STRATEGIES, TECHNIQUES, APPROACHES to CRITICAL THINKING

A Clinical Reasoning Workbook for Nurses

6TH EDITION

STRATEGIES, TECHNIQUES, & APPROACHES TO CRITICAL THINKING

A Clinical Reasoning Workbook for Nurses

Sandra Luz Martinez de Castillo, EdD, RN

Nursing Faculty
Contra Costa College
San Pablo, California

ELSEVIER

ELSEVIER

3251 Riverport Lane
St. Louis, Missouri 63043

STRATEGIES, TECHNIQUES, & APPROACHES TO
CRITICAL THINKING: A CLINICAL REASONING WORKBOOK
FOR NURSES, SIXTH EDITION   ISBN: 978-0-323-44675-4

Notices

Knowledge and best practice in this field are constantly changing. As new research and experience broaden our understanding, changes in research methods, professional practices, or medical treatment may become necessary.

Practitioners and researchers must always rely on their own experience and knowledge in evaluating and using any information, methods, compounds, or experiments described herein. In using such information or methods they should be mindful of their own safety and the safety of others, including parties for whom they have a professional responsibility.

With respect to any drug or pharmaceutical products identified, readers are advised to check the most current information provided (i) on procedures featured or (ii) by the manufacturer of each product to be administered, to verify the recommended dose or formula, the method and duration of administration, and contraindications. It is the responsibility of practitioners, relying on their own experience and knowledge of their patients, to make diagnoses, to determine dosages and the best treatment for each individual patient, and to take all appropriate safety precautions.

To the fullest extent of the law, neither the Publisher nor the authors, contributors, or editors, assume any liability for any injury and/or damage to persons or property as a matter of products liability, negligence or otherwise, or from any use or operation of any methods, products, instructions, or ideas contained in the material herein.

Executive Content Strategist: Lee Henderson
Content Development Manager: Billie Sharp
Content Development Specialist: Sarah Vora/Charlene Ketchum
Publishing Services Manager: Deepthi Unni
Senior Project Manager: Umarani Natarajan
Design Direction: Brian Salisbury

Printed in the United States of America

Last digit is the print number: 9 8 7 6 5 4 3 2 1

Working together
to grow libraries in
developing countries

www.elsevier.com • www.bookaid.org

TO THE STUDENT

Dear Nursing Student,

Congratulations on choosing this wonderful profession. From a practical point of view, nursing is a profession that requires a strong knowledge base, the use of critical thinking skills, professional communication, collaborative practice, and lifelong learning. From a personal point of view, nursing embodies caring. Your clinical experiences will challenge your knowledge and touch your heart!

This workbook is divided into seven sections that consist of clinical situations found in clinical practice. Each section is specifically designed to assist you in developing critical thinking and decision making skills important in clinical practice.

Section One focuses on building your knowledge base and applying this knowledge to short, clinically based patient care situations. The clinical situations in Section One have three purposes: (1) to build your knowledge base and reinforce fundamental concepts and principles, (2) to demonstrate how learned knowledge is applied to clinical situations, and (3) to use critical thinking and clinical reasoning skills as you apply the Critical Thinking Model to the clinical situations presented. Remember that knowledge is fundamental to effectively using critical thinking skills and in promoting clinical reasoning. Get actively involved in the knowledge building learning activities and solicit input from your instructor.

Section Two presents common clinical situations that will help you prioritize selected nursing interventions and make clinical decisions based on sound clinical reasoning. This section introduces you to the SBAR handoff report format and presents progressive clinical situations that allow you to observe how nurses need to constantly assess and reevaluate patient care situations. The nursing process is included in this section to assist you with applying the components of assessment, nursing diagnosis, planning, and implementation.

Section Three presents clinical situations using electronic medical record screens. You are asked to analyze and interpret the data based on the presenting clinical situation and to use the information found in the electronic medical record screens, such as: the Medication Administration Record, Intake and Output Record, Nursing Notes, and the Physician's History and Physical. This activity helps you to (1) focus on gathering the data, and (2) synthesize and make relevant connections between the data.

Section Four focuses on the development of management and leadership skills. As you begin to work with peers and delegate to staff, work-related issues and personnel situations will arise. As with the patient care clinical situations, it is important to apply critical thinking skills as you work through the various clinical situations. Take time to discuss the clinical situation with your peers and focus on your management and leadership skills. Do you have a preferred style of management or leadership?

Section Five provides additional test questions for practice with selecting the most appropriate answer and making nursing decisions based on the clinical situation. You will draw from your knowledge base and your clinical experience as a nursing student to answer the test questions. Review and discuss your rationales to increase your comprehension and knowledge base.

Section Six presents situations that will assist you to apply leadership and delegation skills. The clinical situations offer an opportunity to discuss the scope of practice of the registered nurse, the licensed vocational nurse, and unlicensed personnel as they relate to the situation. In addition, you will experience solving realistic work-related issues encountered in clinical practice.

Section Seven provides you with the opportunity to use reference books and the Internet to research drugs while learning their side effects, or adverse effects. Based on your research findings, it is important for you to compare and contrast drug information and further relate this information to patient teaching and follow-up care.

In addition, the following icons can be found throughout the text to highlight important aspects of practice for nurses. The Teamwork and Collaboration icon ⚙, Safety icon ⚠, and the Patient-Centered Care icon ⚐ highlight where important principles related to QSEN and IPEC are practiced. The Delegation/Supervision icon ☑ highlights selected test questions and clinical situations that require you to consider the functions and duties of licensed and unlicensed personnel and to make a decision that promotes patient safety. The Interprofessional Collaboration icon **IP** highlights test questions and situations that require you to consider the importance of cultivating and maintaining professional relationships with colleagues, patients, and their families.

As you progress through the scenarios, I hope that your knowledge base and critical thinking skills increase and that your nursing school experience is filled with joy.

Dr. Sandra Luz Martinez de Castillo

DEDICATION

To God for this wonderful journey. To Richard, my husband, for his patience and understanding during the preparation of this edition and always to my parents, Blanca and Miguel.

REVIEWERS

Carisa Atkins, MSN, RN
Associate Professor
Associate Nursing Degree
Moberly Area Community College
Moberly, Missouri

Kathleen N. Krov, PhD, CNM, RN, CNE
Professor
Health Science Education – Nursing
Raritan Valley Community College
Branchburg, New Jersey

Elizabeth A. Summers, MSN, RN, CNE
Coordinator of Practical Nursing Program
Department of Practical Nursing
Cass Career Center
Harrisonville, Missouri

Nancy Wiseman, MSN, RN
Nursing Educator
Department of Nursing
Saline County Career Center
Marshall, Missouri

ACKNOWLEDGMENT

To the Elsevier staff, especially Sarah, for their time and dedication to the publication of this edition. To the students, patients, and families who have enriched my life.

CONTENTS

Section Three — Critical Thinking Model Application

Section Four — Management and Leadership

Section Five — NCLEX Examination Preparation

Section Six — Professional Nursing Practice

Section Seven — Evaluation

SECTION 1

Knowledge Application

1-1 PROFESSIONAL NURSING PRACTICE

Fill in the blanks with the requested information:

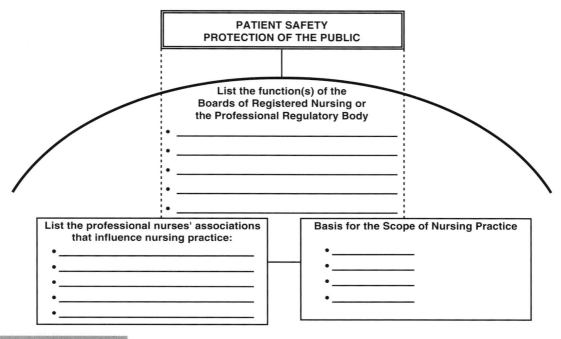

PATIENT SAFETY PROTECTION OF THE PUBLIC

List the function(s) of the Boards of Registered Nursing or the Professional Regulatory Body

- _____
- _____
- _____
- _____
- _____

List the professional nurses' associations that influence nursing practice:

- _____
- _____
- _____
- _____
- _____

Basis for the Scope of Nursing Practice

- _____
- _____
- _____
- _____

CLINICAL SITUATION A student nurse started clinical practice in the acute care setting. The assignment includes caring for a client who will be transferred to a skilled nursing facility today but needs morning care, bathing, and assistance with feeding before discharge. The client also has an indwelling urinary catheter.

Pertinent Terminology	Definition
Nurse Practice Act	_____
Scope of Nursing Practice	_____
	_____
	_____
	_____
Independent Nursing Functions	_____
Dependent Nursing Functions	_____
Interdependent Nursing Functions	_____
	_____
	_____
	_____

From the clinical situation, identify the type of nursing function for the following interventions:

Assigned Nursing Care	Function
Morning care, bathing, feeding, indwelling urinary catheter care	☐ Independent ☐ Dependent ☐ Interdependent

The family arrives and asks whether their father will be transferred to the skilled facility with the urinary catheter. The student consults with the RN, who says that "it should probably be removed."

Assigned Nursing Care	Function
Urinary catheter removal	☐ Independent ☐ Dependent ☐ Interdependent

The RN and the student return to the client's room. The RN is getting ready to administer the morning medications to the client.

Assigned Nursing Care	Function
Administration of medication	☐ Independent ☐ Dependent ☐ Interdependent

The RN is caring for another patient who had abdominal surgery 3 days ago. The patient asks the RN when the urinary catheter is to be removed. The nurse refers to the standard protocol for urinary catheter removal for postoperative patients that is approved by the agency.

Assigned Nursing Care	Function
Urinary catheter removal postoperative based on standard protocol	☐ Independent ☐ Dependent ☐ Interdependent

Collaborative Learning Activity: With a partner, connect to website of the State Board of Registered Nursing or the professional regulatory body for your state and review the regulations governing the scope of practice for the following situations.

1. What is the position of the State Board of Registered Nursing or the professional regulatory body of the state regarding services provided by student nurses?
2. What is the position of the State Board of Registered Nursing or the professional regulatory body of the state regarding delegation of tasks?

1-2 VITAL SIGNS

List the common routes for taking a **temperature**:

1. _____

2. _____

3. _____

4. _____

5. _____

The **blood pressure** may be auscultated in the

_____ and _____ spaces.

Use the diagram to identify the **pulse sites** in the body.

CLINICAL SITUATION   An adult male client has been having a high fever for 2 days. At the physician's office he was found to be febrile. Additionally, the client is complaining of chills, night sweats, anorexia, and fatigue. He is admitted to the hospital. The physician's orders include vital signs (VS) every 4 hours. On admission he had pyrexia. The admission VS are T 102.4°F, P 96, R 26, BP 148/88, pulse ox 98%, pain level 0.

Pertinent Terminology	Definition
Vital Signs	_____
	_____
Temperature	_____
Pulse	_____
Respiration	_____
Pulse Oximetry (Pulse Ox)	_____
	_____
Blood Pressure	_____
Febrile	_____
Pyrexia	_____
Anorexia	_____
Fatigue	_____

From the clinical situation, record today's date and the 0800 admission VS using the following **Graphic Sheet**. Enter the following vital signs for today:

1200	T 103.6°F,	P 108,	R 32,	BP 160/76,	Pulse ox 97%,	Pain level 0
1600	T 101.2°F,	P 98,	R 28,	BP 154/82,	Pulse ox 96%,	Pain level 2
2000	T 100.0°F,	P 80,	R 24,	BP 150/90,	Pulse ox 98%,	Pain level 2

Record the 0800 VS for the next day: T 99.6°F, P 72, R 18, BP 146/94, Pulse ox 97%, and Pain level 0

Draw a line between the temperature recordings to create a graph.

GRAPHIC SHEET

Date												
Time	0400	0800	1200	1600	2000	2400	0400	0800	1200	1600	2000	2400
40°C 104°F												
39.4°C 103°F												
38.9°C 102°F												
38.3°C 101°F												
37.7°C 100°F												
37.2°C 99°F												
37 36.6°C 98°F												
36.1°C 97°F												
35.5°C 96°F												
Pulse												
Resp.												
B/P												
SpO$_2$												

Collaborative Learning Activity: With a partner, identify the normal range(s) for the VS in the adult.

Body temperature   **Oral**   _____

Axillary   _____

_____

Rectal   _____

_____

Tympanic   _____

Pulse   _____

Respirations   _____

Blood pressure   _____

Pulse oximetry   _____

Pain assessment   _____

1-3 TEMPERATURE

The **body temperature** is regulated through the

_____.

Body temperature remains constant through **heat production** and **heat loss**.

Factors that influence heat production:

- _____
- _____

Factors that influence heat loss:

- _____
- _____
- _____
- _____

Body temperature is affected by:

1. _____

2. _____

3. _____

4. _____

5. _____

6. _____

CLINICAL SITUATION A 79-year-old client was brought to the emergency department after having fainted while sitting outside at a family gathering. The physician admitted the client with the diagnosis of heatstroke. On admission the vital signs are T 40.5°C, P 100, R 26, BP 118/64. The client's skin is flushed and feels hot and dry. The client is awake and denies pain but is complaining of nausea. The physician orders the temperature to be monitored every 2 hours.

Pertinent Terminology	Definition
Temperature	_____
Core Temperature	_____
	_____
Hyperthermia	_____
Hypothermia	_____
Heatstroke	_____
	_____
Conduction	_____
	_____
Convection	_____
Evaporation	_____
Radiation	_____

From the clinical situation, explain how the **evaporation factor initially** acts to prevent the client from developing heatstroke:

_____

Electronic temperature recordings found in the patient's electronic health record (EHR)

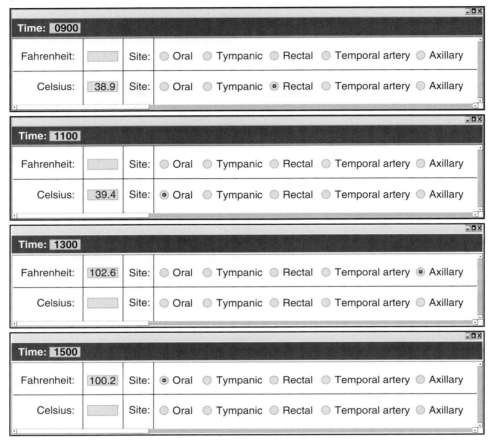

Collaborative Learning Activity: **Graph** the above EHR temperature readings on the Temperature Recording Sheet. Draw a line between each temperature recording. Compare your **Temperature Recording Sheet** with that of a partner.

TEMPERATURE RECORDING SHEET

Time	0800	0900	1000	1100	1200	1300	1400	1500
40.5°C 105°F								
40°C 104°F								
39.4°C 103°F								
38.9°C 102°F								
38.3°C 101°F								
37.7°C 100°F								
37.2°C 99°F								
37 36.6°C 98°F								
36.1°C 97°F								
35.5°C 96°F								

APPLYING CRITICAL THINKING TO TEST QUESTIONS

INSTRUCTIONS: Circle the one best answer for each test question. Write your rationale for selecting the answer. To enhance your learning and test-taking skills, discuss your answer and rationale with a partner. The answer and the rationale can be found on the back of this page.

1. The nurse is using an electronic thermometer to take an oral temperature. After taking the oral temperature, the nurse obtains a reading of 94.2°F. Which follow-up action is most appropriate for the nurse to do?
   a. Use another electronic thermometer to retake the temperature.
   b. Feel the client's skin temperature.
   c. Take a rectal temperature.
   d. Record the findings.

   Rationale for your selection: _____
   _____
   _____
   _____
   _____

2. Which statement is most accurate regarding the body temperature measurement?
   a. An oral temperature reading of 98.6°F is the most normal temperature for adults.
   b. A rectal temperature reading of 100°F indicates that the client is febrile.
   c. A core temperature reading is the most accurate indicator of the body temperature.
   d. Temporal artery temperature measurements are most accurately performed by the RN.

   Rationale for your selection: _____
   _____
   _____
   _____
   _____

3. The nurse is caring for a client who has an oral temperature of 99.6°F at 8:00 AM, the start of the day shift. The client's care plan indicates that vital signs should be taken once a shift. In planning care for the client, which action is most appropriate?
   a. Ensure that the temperature is taken promptly at 4:00 PM.
   b. Call the physician for a more frequent order.
   c. Take the temperature as necessary.
   d. Begin cooling measures.

   Rationale for your selection: _____
   _____
   _____
   _____
   _____

ANSWER KEY FOR
APPLYING CRITICAL THINKING SKILLS TO TEST QUESTIONS

HELPFUL HINTS: Read all test questions carefully. Identify key words in the question that will guide you in answering the question. In these test questions the **key words** to consider are **"follow-up"** and **"most appropriate."** Compare your rationale with the one in the test question.

1. The nurse is using an electronic thermometer to take an oral temperature. After taking the oral temperature, the nurse obtains a reading of 94.2°F. Which follow-up action is most appropriate for the nurse to do?
   (a.) Use another electronic thermometer to retake the temperature.
   b. Feel the client's skin temperature.
   c. Take a rectal temperature.
   d. Record the findings.

   Rationale: The answer is (a). Because the nurse is using an electronic thermometer, it is important for the nurse to ensure that the equipment is functioning. The temperature recording is low and should be taken again. Option (b) does not provide the most accurate information, and (c) is not appropriate; option (d) should be done after the temperature is verified.

2. Which statement is most accurate regarding the body temperature measurement?
   a. An oral temperature reading of 98.6°F is the most normal temperature for adults.
   b. A rectal temperature reading of 100°F indicates that the client is febrile.
   (c.) A core temperature reading is the most accurate indicator of the body temperature.
   d. Temporal artery temperature measurements are most accurately performed by the RN.

   Rationale: The answer is (c). The core body temperature refers to the internal parts of our body, such as vital organs such as the heart, liver, kidneys, and the blood itself, and is regulated by the hypothalamus. Options (a) and (b) identify a single temperature measurement. It is important to recall the average temperature range and that surface temperature may fluctuate throughout the day. Option (d), the temporal artery temperature, may be taken by nurse assistive personnel.

3. The nurse is caring for a client who has an oral temperature of 99.6°F at 8:00 AM, the start of the day shift. The client's care plan indicates that vital signs should be taken once a shift. In planning care for the client, which action is most appropriate?
   a. Ensure that the temperature is taken promptly at 4:00 PM.
   b. Call the physician for a more frequent order.
   (c.) Take the temperature as necessary.
   d. Begin cooling measures.

   Rationale: The answer is (c). The nurse can make an independent decision to take the temperature more frequently to ensure safe nursing care. Option (a) does not allow for a thorough, ongoing assessment. Options (b) and (d) are not necessary at this time.

1-4 PULSE

The normal **pulse rate range** for an adult is

_____.

The **pulse characteristics** include a description

of the _____, _____, and

_____ of the pulse.

The **pulse** is affected by:

1. _____

2. _____

3. _____

4. _____

5. _____

6. _____

7. _____

8. _____

Draw circles on the diagram that identify the sites where the **pulse** is found in the body.

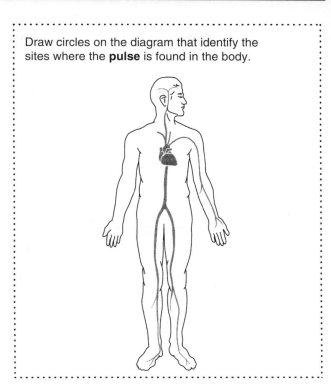

CLINICAL SITUATION A 52-year-old male client has been complaining of a rapid heartbeat. He says that it feels as if his "heart is racing." His wife took him to the urgent care clinic where he was found to have an irregular pulse of 160 bpm; he was transferred to the hospital. On admission to the hospital his vital signs are T 98.4°F, P 168, R 28, BP 146/90, denies pain. His skin is moist, and he is very anxious. The physician orders the administration of cardiac medications and orders the pulse to be monitored every 2 hours.

Pertinent Terminology	Definition
Pulse	_____
	_____
Peripheral Pulse	_____
Apical Pulse	_____
Stroke Volume	_____
Cardiac Output	_____
	_____
Pulse Rhythm	_____
Pulse Quality	_____
Tachycardia	_____
Bradycardia	_____
Arrhythmia	_____
Pulse Deficit	_____

From the clinical situation, use the admission pulse of 168 bpm to assist in identifying the words in the parentheses that would **best describe** the characteristics of this pulse:

Pulse Characteristic	Descriptive Words	Selected Word(s)
Rate	(rapid, tachycardia, bradycardia, increased)	
Rhythm	(regular, irregular, abnormal, dysrhythmia)	
Quality	(weak, thready, bounding, difficult to palpate)	

Collaborative Learning Activity: With a partner, identify the pulse site in each diagram and write in the reason for checking the pulse from this area.

Pulse: _____

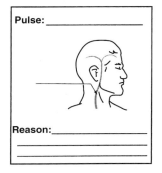

Reason:_____
_____
_____

Pulse:_____

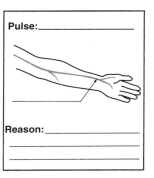

Reason:_____
_____

Pulse: _____

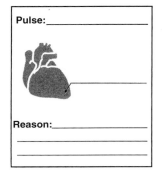

Reason:_____
_____
_____

Pulse:_____

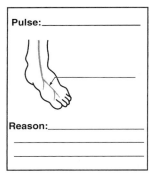

Reason:_____
_____
_____

The **apical pulse** is taken when _____
_____
_____

To take an **apical pulse**, the stethoscope is placed on _____
_____

APPLYING CRITICAL THINKING SKILLS TO TEST QUESTIONS

INSTRUCTIONS: Circle the one best answer for each test question. Write your rationale for selecting the answer. To enhance your learning and test-taking skills, discuss your answer and rationale with a partner. The answer and the rationale can be found on the back of this page.

1. The nurse describes the radial pulse as "thready and irregular" after taking morning vital signs. The most appropriate follow-up nursing action is to:
   a. notify the physician.
   b. check the apical pulse.
   c. record the pulse.
   d. check the previous pulse.

   Rationale for your selection: _____
   _____
   _____
   _____
   _____
   _____

2. The nurse is auscultating the apical pulse on a client. In counting the apical pulse, the nurse counts:
   a. each lub-dub as one beat.
   b. each lub-dub as two beats.
   c. the pulse for 10 seconds and multiplies by 6.
   d. the pulse for 30 seconds and multiplies by 2.

   Rationale for your selection: _____
   _____
   _____
   _____
   _____
   _____

3. The nurse is instructed to check for a pedal pulse on a client at the beginning of the shift. To carry out this intervention, it is most appropriate for the nurse to:
   a. count the brachial pulse for 30 seconds.
   b. count the posterior tibial pulse for 1 full minute.
   c. palpate for the dorsalis pedis.
   d. palpate for the popliteal pulse.

   Rationale for your selection: _____
   _____
   _____
   _____
   _____
   _____

ANSWER KEY FOR
APPLYING CRITICAL THINKING SKILLS TO TEST QUESTIONS

HELPFUL HINTS: Read all test questions carefully. Identify key words in the question that will guide you in answering the question. In these test questions the **key words** to consider are **"most appropriate."** Compare your rationale with the one in the test question.

1. The nurse describes the radial pulse as "thready and irregular" after taking morning vital signs. The most appropriate follow-up nursing action is to:
   a. notify the physician.
   (b.) check the apical pulse.
   c. record the pulse.
   d. check the previous pulse.

   Rationale: The answer is (b). It is the nurse's responsibility to validate abnormal findings. Therefore the most appropriate follow-up action in this question is to check the apical pulse. This will assist the nurse to fully assess the findings. Although options (a), (c), and (d) are all actions that the nurse would do, they are not the most appropriate for this situation.

2. The nurse is auscultating the apical pulse on a client. In counting the apical pulse, the nurse counts:
   (a.) each lub-dub as one beat.
   b. each lub-dub as two beats.
   c. the pulse for 10 seconds and multiplies by 6.
   d. the pulse for 30 seconds and multiplies by 2.

   Rationale: The answer is (a). Each lub represents the closure of the mitral and tricuspid valves during systole and the dub represents the closure of the aortic and pulmonic valves during diastole. Together the lub-dub sounds are counted as one beat. Options (b), (c), and (d) do not describe the correct technique for counting the apical pulse.

3. The nurse is instructed to check for a pedal pulse on a client at the beginning of the shift. To carry out this intervention, it is most appropriate for the nurse to:
   a. count the brachial pulse for 30 seconds.
   b. count the posterior tibial pulse for 1 full minute.
   (c.) palpate for the dorsalis pedis.
   d. palpate for the popliteal pulse.

   Rationale: The answer is (c). This question addresses the nurse's understanding of pedal pulses. Therefore in this situation, it is most appropriate for the nurse to locate and palpate the pulse in the feet. Although option (b) identifies one of the pedal pulses, it is not necessary to take a pedal pulse for a full minute. Options (a) and (d) are not appropriate in carrying out this nursing order.

1-5 RESPIRATION

The normal respiratory rate range for an adult is _____.

The **characteristics of respiration** include a description of the _____, _____, and _____ of the respirations.

The factors that affect the **characteristics of respiration** include:

1. _____
2. _____
3. _____
4. _____
5. _____
6. _____
7. _____
8. _____
9. _____
10. _____

A **normal** respiratory pattern consists of a full inspiration and a full expiration counted over one minute as the diagram illustrates:

One minute

Exp.

Insp.

The diagram demonstrates a _____ respiratory pattern.

One minute

Exp.

Insp.

The diagram demonstrates a _____ respiratory pattern.

CLINICAL SITUATION A male client has been a smoker for 20 years. He has noticed increased shortness of breath (SOB) for the past 6 months and is complaining of a productive cough with thick whitish phlegm. The nurse notices that his respiratory rate is 32 and regular and describes his lung sounds as fine crackling sounds heard on inspiration. Pulse oximetry is 92% on room air.

Pertinent Terminology	Definition
Respiration	_____
Tachypnea	_____
Bradypnea	_____
Eupnea	_____
Apnea	_____
Orthopnea	_____
	_____
Dyspnea	_____
Cheyne-Stokes	_____
	_____
Kussmaul	_____
	_____
Phlegm	_____

From the clinical situation, use the respiratory rate of 32 to assist in identifying the words in the parentheses that would **best describe** the characteristics of this respiratory pattern:

Respiratory Characteristic	Descriptive Words	Selected Word(s)
Rate	(eupnea, tachypnea, bradypnea, apnea)	
Depth	(deep, full inspiration/expiration, short, shallow)	
Rhythm	(regular, irregular)	

Draw a line to match the **identified lung sounds** below with the appropriate description. (Visit www.evolve.elsevier.com/castillo to hear sample lung sounds.)

Wheeze   crackling sound, may be fine or coarse, heard frequently on inspiration

Crackle   coarse, harsh, loud sound, best heard on expiration

Gurgle   continuous high-pitched musical sound best heard on expiration

Circle the lung sound that best describes the client's lung sounds.

Collaborative Learning Activity: Draw a diagram that represents the respiratory pattern identified under each box. Compare and discuss your diagrams with a partner.

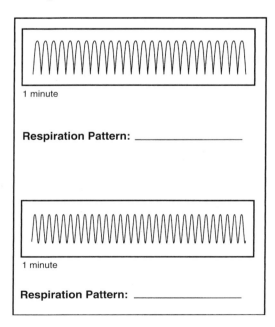

1 minute

Respiration Pattern: _____

1 minute

Respiration Pattern: _____

1 minute

Respiration Pattern: _____

1 minute

Respiration Pattern: _____

APPLYING CRITICAL THINKING SKILLS TO TEST QUESTIONS

INSTRUCTIONS: Circle the best answer for each test question. Write your rationale for selecting the answer. To enhance your learning and test-taking skills, discuss your answer and rationale with a partner. The answer and the rationale can be found on the back of this page.

1. The nurse is taking the vital signs of a client who has shortness of breath. In counting the respiratory rate it is most important for the nurse to:
   a. observe the rise and fall of the chest for 15 seconds.
   b. assess the respiratory pattern for 30 seconds.
   c. sit the client in a semi-Fowler's position.
   d. count the respiratory rate for 1 minute.

   Rationale for your selection: _____
   _____
   _____
   _____
   _____
   _____

2. The nurse assesses the respiratory rate of an adult client to be 20 and unlabored. The most appropriate follow-up nursing intervention is to:
   a. reassess the respiratory rate.
   b. record the findings.
   c. check the pulse oximeter.
   d. place the client in high Fowler's position.

   Rationale for your selection: _____
   _____
   _____
   _____
   _____
   _____

3. The physician orders pulse oximetry checks on the client once a shift. To effectively use the pulse oximeter on the client, the nurse would:
   a. place the pulse oximeter on the client's finger and wait for a reading.
   b. give the client oxygen before using the pulse oximeter.
   c. place the client in high Fowler's position.
   d. use the pulse oximeter only when the client has dyspnea.

   Rationale for your selection: _____
   _____
   _____
   _____
   _____
   _____

ANSWER KEY FOR
APPLYING CRITICAL THINKING SKILLS TO TEST QUESTIONS

HELPFUL HINTS: Read all test questions carefully. Identify key words in the question that will guide you in answering the question. In these test questions the **key words** to consider are **"most important," "most appropriate,"** and **"effectively use."** Compare your rationale with the one found for each question.

1. The nurse is taking the vital signs of a client who has shortness of breath. In counting the respiratory rate it is most important for the nurse to:
   a. observe the rise and fall of the chest for 15 seconds.
   b. assess the respiratory pattern for 30 seconds.
   c. sit the client in a semi-Fowler's position.
   d. count the respiratory rate for 1 minute.

   Rationale: The answer is (d). Because the client has shortness of breath, it is most important for the nurse to fully assess the respirations for 1 minute. Option (a) does not allow the nurse to fully assess the respiratory pattern; option (b), assessment of an abnormal respiratory pattern, should be done for 1 full minute; and option (c) compromises the respiratory system. _____
   _____
   _____
   _____

2. The nurse assesses the respiratory rate of an adult client to be 20 and unlabored. The most appropriate follow-up nursing intervention is to:
   a. reassess the respiratory rate.
   b. record the findings.
   c. check the pulse oximeter.
   d. place the client in high Fowler's position.

   Rationale: The answer is (b). The findings are normal; therefore, the next nursing intervention is to record the findings. Options (a), (c), and (d) can be performed if the nurse assesses an abnormal rate. _____
   _____
   _____
   _____

3. The physician orders pulse oximetry checks on the client once a shift. To effectively use the pulse oximeter on the client, the nurse would:
   a. place the pulse oximeter on the client's finger and wait for a reading.
   b. give the client oxygen before using the pulse oximeter.
   c. place the client in high Fowler's position.
   d. use the pulse oximeter only when the client has dyspnea.

   Rationale: The answer is (a). The answer describes how to use the pulse oximeter. Options (b) and (c) are incorrect in answering how to effectively use the pulse oximeter. Option (d) is incorrect: a pulse oximeter can be used to assess oxygenation in any client. _____
   _____
   _____
   _____

1-6 BLOOD PRESSURE

The normal blood pressure for an adult is
_____.

Factors that affect blood pressure include:

1. _____
2. _____
3. _____
4. _____
5. _____
6. _____
7. _____
8. _____
9. _____
10. _____

Identify the parts of the following items used in obtaining a blood pressure:

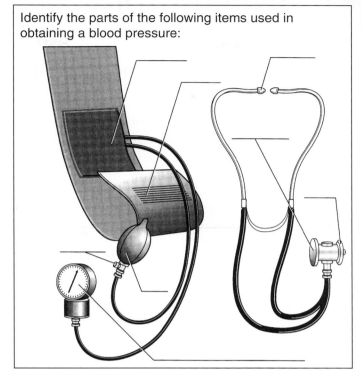

CLINICAL SITUATION   A 65-year-old African American man goes weekly to the hypertension clinic for blood pressure checks. He has a 20-year history of smoking two packs of cigarettes a day. His father died from heart disease and his brother has hypertension. He lives alone, does not get out much, and his diet is mainly pre-made frozen meals or canned foods. His current blood pressure reading is 174/104 mm Hg, and he is complaining of a headache and dizziness when getting up in the morning.

Pertinent Terminology	Definition
Blood Pressure	_____
Systolic Pressure	_____
Diastolic Pressure	_____
Korotkoff Sounds	_____
	_____
Pulse Pressure	_____
Prehypertension	_____
Hypertension	_____
Hypotension	_____
	_____
Orthostatic Hypotension	_____
	_____
Auscultatory Gap	_____
	_____

From the clinical situation, identify the **factors** that predisposed the patient to the development of hypertension:

_____   _____   _____

_____   _____   _____

Collaborative Learning Activity: The clinic nurse monitors the patient's blood pressure for 2 days (11/1, 11/2) and documents the blood pressure recordings in the patient's electronic health record.

	Date: 11/1 Time: 1100	Date: 11/1 Time: 1130		
Systolic	160	156	Site	☐ right wrist ☐ left wrist ☑ upper right arm ☐ upper left arm ☑ brachial ☐ upper right thigh ☐ upper left thigh
Diastolic	100	98	Position	☑ Lying ☐ Sitting ☐ Standing
			Device	☑ Automated ☐ Small Adult cuff ☐ Adult cuff ☐ Large Adult cuff ☐ Adult Thigh cuff

	Date: 11/2 Time: 1100		
Systolic	170	Site	☐ upper right arm ☑ upper left arm ☑ brachial ☐ upper right thigh ☐ upper left thigh
Diastolic	90	Position	☑ Lying ☐ Sitting ☐ Standing
		Device	☐ Automated ☐ Small Adult cuff ☑ Adult cuff ☐ Large Adult cuff ☐ Adult Thigh cuff

	Date: 11/2 Time: 1102		
Systolic	164	Site	☐ upper right arm ☑ upper left arm ☑ brachial ☐ upper right thigh ☐ upper left thigh
Diastolic	90	Position	☐ Lying ☑ Sitting ☐ Standing
		Device	☐ Automated ☐ Small Adult cuff ☑ Adult cuff ☐ Large Adult cuff ☐ Adult Thigh cuff

	Date: 11/2 Time: 1105		
Systolic	140	Site	☐ upper right arm ☑ upper left arm ☑ brachial ☐ upper right thigh ☐ upper left thigh
Diastolic	86	Position	☐ Lying ☐ Sitting ☑ Standing
		Device	☐ Automated ☐ Small Adult cuff ☑ Adult cuff ☐ Large Adult cuff ☐ Adult Thigh cuff

Based on the blood pressure recordings of the second day, with a partner identify and discuss safety concerns for the patient.

_____

_____

_____

APPLYING CRITICAL THINKING SKILLS TO TEST QUESTIONS

INSTRUCTIONS: Circle the one best answer for each test question. Write your rationale for selecting the answer. To enhance your learning and test-taking skills, discuss your answer and rationale with a partner. The answer and the rationale can be found on the back of this page.

1. The nurse is preparing to take the blood pressure of an adult patient for the first time. After placing the cuff on the patient's upper arm, it is most important for the nurse to:
   a. wait 1 minute before taking the blood pressure.
   b. place the stethoscope at the antecubital space.
   c. inflate the cuff to 150 mm Hg.
   d. palpate the systolic pressure.

   Rationale for your selection: _____
   _____
   _____
   _____
   _____
   _____

2. The nurse uses a Doppler device to obtain the blood pressure measurement. In documenting the findings, the nurse will record the:
   a. systolic measurement.
   b. systolic and diastolic measurements.
   c. diastolic measurement.
   d. auscultatory gap.

   Rationale for your selection: _____
   _____
   _____
   _____
   _____
   _____

3. In which of the following clients would the nurse expect a decreased blood pressure? A client:
   a. who is very anxious about being in the hospital.
   b. scheduled for major surgery.
   c. with a severe head injury.
   d. who hemorrhaged after surgery.

   Rationale for your selection: _____
   _____
   _____
   _____
   _____
   _____

1 Knowledge Application

ANSWER KEY FOR
APPLYING CRITICAL THINKING SKILLS TO TEST QUESTIONS

HELPFUL HINTS: Read all test questions carefully. Identify key words in the question that will guide you in answering the question. In these test questions the key words to consider are **"first time," "initial action,"** and **"most appropriate."** Compare your rationale with the one in the test question.

1. The nurse is preparing to take the blood pressure of an adult patient for the first time. After placing the cuff on the patient's upper arm, it is most important for the nurse to:
   a. wait 1 minute before taking the blood pressure.
   b. place the stethoscope at the antecubital space.
   c. inflate the cuff to 150 mm Hg.
   d. palpate the systolic pressure.

   Rationale: The answer is (d). Palpating for the systolic pressure provides the nurse with information for inflating the cuff to ensure an accurate systolic reading. Although option (b) is an action that the nurse would do, it is not the initial action. Options (a) and (c) are not appropriate for this situation.

2. The nurse uses a Doppler device to obtain the blood pressure measurement. In documenting the findings, the nurse will record the:
   a. systolic measurement.
   b. systolic and diastolic measurements.
   c. diastolic measurement.
   d. auscultatory gap.

   Rationale: The answer is (a). Doppler devices amplify sound. In finding the blood pressure, only the systolic measurement can be obtained with the use of a Doppler device. Options (b), (c), and (d) are not possible options when using a Doppler device.

3. In which of the following clients would the nurse expect a decreased blood pressure? A client:
   a. who is very anxious about being in the hospital.
   b. scheduled for major surgery.
   c. with a severe head injury.
   d. who hemorrhaged after surgery.

   Rationale: The answer is (d). Conditions that decrease the blood volume also decrease the cardiac output, which contributes to a decrease in blood pressure. Options (a), (b), and (c) are conditions that cause vasoconstriction, which increases the blood pressure.

1-7 PAIN ASSESSMENT

Pain is the _____ vital sign.

Assessment of the patient's pain is done:

_____

_____

_____

Common behaviors that may indicate that the patient is experiencing pain include:

1. _____

2. _____

3. _____

4. _____

5. _____

List **words** frequently used by patients to describe the quality of the pain sensation.

CLINICAL SITUATION   Patient A is a 27-year-old male who sustained a sprained left ankle 2 days ago after tripping and falling while playing basketball.

Patient B is a 56-year-old female who is diagnosed with bone cancer and is admitted to the hospital for chemotherapy.

Patient C is a 79-year-old female who had a right hip replacement 2 days ago. She continues to demonstrate disorientation to time and place as noted on admission to the hospital. However, the handoff report indicates that she showed signs of increased restlessness during the night and this morning.

Pertinent Terminology	Definition
Pain	_____ _____
Acute Pain	_____ _____
Chronic Pain **Breakthrough Pain**	_____ _____
Cancer Pain	_____ _____
Pain Threshold **Pain Tolerance**	_____ _____
Pain Assessment Tool	_____ _____

UNIDIMENSIONAL PAIN ASSESSMENT SCALES

Visit *www.evolve.elsevier.com/castillo* to access the various pain assessment scales. **Select the most appropriate pain scale** for the patients in the clinical situation.

- For Patient A, the _____ pain assessment scale is appropriate for the nurse to use.
- For Patient B, the _____ pain assessment scale is appropriate for the nurse to use.
- For Patient C, the _____ assessment scales are appropriate for the nurse to use.

Use the clinical situation and these follow-up assessments to make clinical decisions that focus on **patient-centered care** and **pain management**.

On assessing Patient A at 0800, the patient reports a pain level of 5. The swelling from the left ankle has remained the same since the injury. His pain medication is ordered q4h and the last dose was given at 0415. The most appropriate follow-up is to _____

_____

On assessing Patient B at 0815, the patient reports a pain level of 9. The patient has a PCA with continuous morphine sulfate infusion. Morphine sulfate 3 mg is ordered q2h direct IV injection for breakthrough pain. It was last given at 0530. The most appropriate follow-up is to _____

_____

On assessing Patient C at 0745, the nurse finds the patient restless, grabbing at her bed linens, and pulling on her right hip dressing. The nurse is unable to obtain a verbal pain level from the patient. The most appropriate follow-up is to _____

_____

Collaborative Learning Activity: With a partner, read and evaluate the following statements. Decide whether the statement is True or False. For each statement, provide a rationale that supports your clinical decision.

Statement	True	False	Rationale to Support Your Clinical Decision
Changes in pulse, respirations, and blood pressure are strong indicators of the intensity of pain experienced by the patient.			
Older adults report pain less often.			
Self-report of pain level is the most reliable method to assess pain intensity.			

1-8 BODY MECHANICS

List the **factors** that affect a patient's ability to move and maintain body alignment:

1. _____
2. _____
3. _____
4. _____
5. _____
6. _____
7. _____

Use the diagram to identify the **four basic principles** of body mechanics:

1. _____
2. _____
3. _____
4. _____

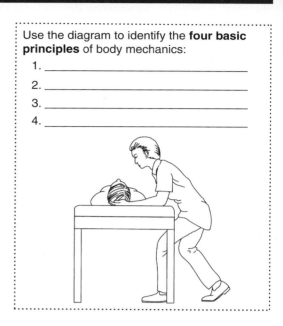

CLINICAL SITUATION   The client has had a cerebral vascular accident (CVA) and as a result has left-sided hemiplegia. The physician orders the client to be out of bed (OOB) twice a day and to be turned every 2 hours while in bed. The RN asks the staff to do passive range of motion (ROM) exercises to the client's left side and to use supportive devices to ensure proper body alignment. The client is to be encouraged to do active ROM to the right side extremities.

Pertinent Terminology	Definition
Range of Motion	_____
Active ROM	_____
Passive ROM	_____
CVA	_____
	_____
Hemiplegia	_____
Alignment	_____
	_____
Hand Roll	_____
Trochanter Roll	_____
	_____
Ankle-Foot Orthotic	_____
Foot Drop	_____
Flaccid	_____

From the clinical situation, **(1) identify** the **major body areas** that would require special nursing care, **(2) select** the most appropriate **supportive device** from the list that will assist in maintaining proper body alignment for the client, and **(3) state the complication** the nursing care will help to prevent.

Hand Roll	Trochanter Roll	Pillow	Trapeze Bar	Ankle-Foot Brace

Major Body Area	Supportive Device	This Helps to Prevent

Select the activities of daily living (ADLs) below that the client can perform **independently** throughout the day that encourage **active ROM** to the **right side** of the body:

- ☐ Brushing teeth
- ☐ Transferring OOB
- ☐ Flexing/extending ankle
- ☐ Combing hair

- ☐ Ambulating
- ☐ Standing
- ☐ Washing face
- ☐ Feeding

Collaborative Learning Activity: With a partner, beginning with number 1, **number the following interventions** in the order necessary to assist the client to transfer from the bed to a wheelchair:

_____ Place wheelchair at a 45-degree angle to the bed.
_____ Lock the wheelchair brakes.
_____ Assist the client to a sitting position at the side of the bed.
_____ Provide instructions to the client.
_____ Cross left lower extremity over right lower extremity.
_____ Have the client pivot toward the wheelchair.
_____ Lower the client into the wheelchair.
_____ Stand the client; support left lower extremity.
_____ Have the client support left upper extremity with right upper extremity.

1-9 HYGIENE

The **purpose of providing a bath** is to:

1. _____
2. _____
3. _____
4. _____
5. _____

Identify the various types of baths:

1. _____
2. _____
3. _____
4. _____
5. _____

Place a "✓" mark on the information that best describes the following:

Early morning care includes:
☐ Starting the bath early in the morning.
☐ Providing/assisting with oral hygiene.
☐ Washing face and hands.
☐ Offering bedpan, urinal, or assistance to the bathroom.

Hour-Before-Sleep care includes:
☐ Providing a back rub for the client.
☐ Straightening the bed linens.
☐ Providing/assisting with oral hygiene.
☐ Taking the vital signs.

CLINICAL SITUATION   An 88-year-old female client has been in the hospital for 2 days with an irregular heartbeat. She is confused and just lies in bed. The RN informs you that the client has urinary and bowel incontinence and is wearing an adult incontinence pad. Her skin is very fragile, she has several ecchymotic areas on the lower extremities, she is wearing antiembolic stockings, and the pneumatic compression stockings are off. Her toenails are long, yellowish, and thick. She has dried feces under her fingernails.

Pertinent Terminology	Definition
Antiembolic Stockings	_____
Pneumatic Compression	_____
Stockings	_____
	_____
Stomatitis	_____
Canthus	_____
Ecchymosis	_____
Perineum	_____
	_____
Labia Majora	_____
Labia Minora	_____
Prepuce	_____

Use the clinical situation to identify the **most appropriate** nursing interventions for taking care of the client's hands and feet. **Circle** the nursing interventions below that you would implement:

IP NURSING INTERVENTIONS

HANDS

1. Do nothing until the RN informs you.
2. Soak the hands in lukewarm water.
3. Give the bath as usual, but do not soak the hands.
4. Use a greenstick or cotton swab to remove the feces.
5. Cut the fingernails carefully to prevent further collection under the nail beds.

FEET

1. Remove the antiembolic stockings during the bath.
2. Clean the feet with lukewarm water.
3. Give a partial bath; apply lotion.
4. Dry well between the toes.
5. Cut the toenails carefully straight across.

Describe the proper method for performing perineal care on a:

Female: _____

_____

Male: _____

_____

Collaborative Learning Activity: With a partner, identify the type of bath **most appropriate** for the following clinical situations:

Clinical Situations	Type of Bath		
A 39-year-old woman who had abdominal surgery 5 days ago and will be discharged this morning	Complete bag bath	Partial self-help	Shower (MD order/ policy)
A 56-year-old patient admitted with lung problems who gets very short of breath with mild exertion	Complete bag bath	Partial	Shower
A 23-year-old woman who is alert but had a grand mal seizure 2 days ago	Complete bag bath	Partial	Shower
A 46-year-old patient who had a motor vehicle accident yesterday, had a mild concussion but no fractures	Complete bag bath	Partial	Shower

1-10 INFECTION CONTROL/TRANSMISSION OF ORGANISMS

Provide examples of the following elements found in the **chain of infection**:

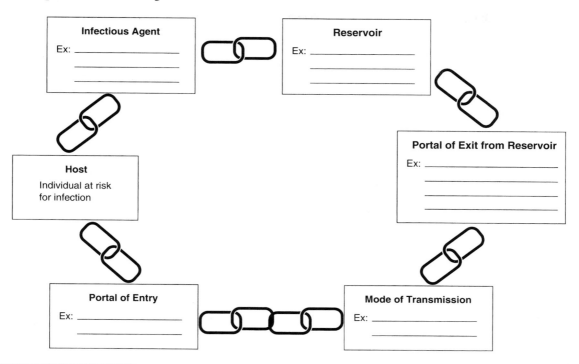

Infectious Agent

Ex: _____
_____
_____

Reservoir

Ex: _____
_____
_____

Portal of Exit from Reservoir

Ex: _____
_____
_____
_____

Host

Individual at risk
for infection

Mode of Transmission

Ex: _____
_____

Portal of Entry

Ex: _____
_____

CLINICAL SITUATION   A young woman has recently begun nursing school. During her second week in the clinical setting, she takes care of a 79-year-old client who was admitted with dehydration. The client has a recent history of shingles and is in the convalescent stage of illness. The client's skin is very dry, and his oral temperature is 100.4°F. His urine is dark amber, and his WBC is 13,000/mm^3.

Pertinent Terminology	Definition
Shingles	_____
Dehydration	_____
Incubation Stage	_____
	_____
Prodromal Stage	_____
	_____
	_____
Illness Stage	_____
	_____
Convalescent Stage	_____
	_____
Asepsis	_____
Nosocomial	_____
Iatrogenic	_____
	_____

From the clinical situation, identify the **factors** that make the client susceptible to getting an infection.

Explain **why** each of the **factors** identified makes the client susceptible to getting an infection.

1. _____
2. _____
3. _____
4. _____

Define medical asepsis: _____
_____

Define surgical asepsis: _____
_____

In caring for the client, the nurse will use _____ asepsis.

Collaborative Learning Activity: With a partner, fill in the diagrams with the proper elements in the chain of infection as it applies to each situation:

   1. A family member who has a cold stops in to visit Mr. Wu.

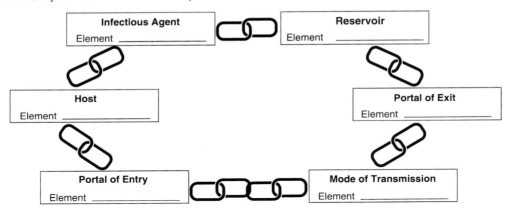

   2. A nursing assistant goes from patient to patient without changing gloves.

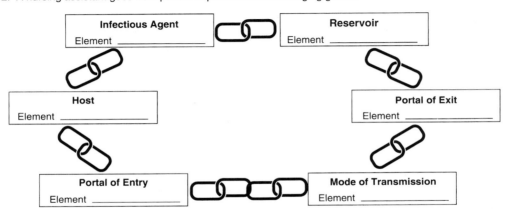

APPLYING CRITICAL THINKING SKILLS TO TEST QUESTIONS

INSTRUCTIONS: Circle the best answer(s) for each test question. Write your rationale for selecting the answer(s). To enhance your learning and test-taking skills, discuss your answer(s) and rationale(s) with a partner. The answer and the rationale can be found on the back of this page.

1. The nurse is taking care of a client who has a respiratory infection with a productive cough. To promote infection control, the nurse is most correct to (Select all that apply.):
   a. use alcohol-based hand rubs.
   b. push oral fluids every shift.
   c. have the client use a tissue when coughing.
   d. auscultate the lung sounds every 4 hours.
   e. hand wash with nonantimicrobial soap and water.

   Rationale for your selection: _____
   _____
   _____
   _____
   _____
   _____

2. The client has been diagnosed with a gastrointestinal bacterium obtained from drinking contaminated water. In the chain of infection, the water is the:
   a. portal of entry.
   b. reservoir.
   c. portal of exit.
   d. infectious agent.

   Rationale for your selection: _____
   _____
   _____
   _____
   _____
   _____

3. The client's abdominal dressing is described as having a moderate amount of serosanguineous drainage and a very foul odor. In planning the dressing change, it is most important for the nurse to:
   a. apply extra dressings to the wound.
   b. use sterile gloves to change the dressing.
   c. wash her hands before and after the dressing change.
   d. change the abdominal dressing more often.

   Rationale for your selection: _____
   _____
   _____
   _____
   _____
   _____

ANSWER KEY FOR
APPLYING CRITICAL THINKING SKILLS TO TEST QUESTIONS

HELPFUL HINTS: Read all test questions carefully. Identify **key words** in the question that will guide you in answering the question. In these test questions the key words to consider are **"most correct,"** and **"most important."** Compare your rationale with the one in the test question.

1. The nurse is taking care of a client who has a respiratory infection with a productive cough. To promote infection control, the nurse is most correct to (Select all that apply.):
   a. use alcohol-based hand rubs. ⊘
   b. push oral fluids every shift.
   c. have the client use a tissue when coughing. ⊘
   d. auscultate the lung sounds every 4 hours.
   e. hand wash with nonantimicrobial soap and water. ⊘

   Rationale: The answers (a), (c), and (e) are infection control principles and practices recommended by the Centers for Disease Control and Prevention to help reduce the transmission of diseases. Options (b) and (d) are good nursing interventions but are not effective in reducing the transmission of diseases.

2. The client has been diagnosed with a gastrointestinal bacterium obtained from drinking contaminated water. In the chain of infection, the water is the:
   a. portal of entry.
   b. reservoir. ⊘
   c. portal of exit.
   d. infectious agent.

   Rationale: The answer is (b). The water is the reservoir that provided the environment for the infectious agent to reproduce. Options (a), (c), and (d) are part of the chain of infection, but the water is the reservoir.

3. The client's abdominal dressing is described as having a moderate amount of serosanguineous drainage and a very foul odor. In planning the dressing change, it is most important for the nurse to:
   a. apply extra dressings to the wound.
   b. use sterile gloves to change the dressing.
   c. wash her hands before and after the dressing change. ⊘
   d. change the abdominal dressing more often.

   Rationale: The answer is (c). Handwashing is the single most effective method in decreasing the spread of pathogens. Option (a) can be done, but it is not the most important option; options (b) and (d) are ordered by the practitioner.

1-11 SKIN INTEGRITY

List the **factors** that increase the **risk** for development of a pressure ulcer:

1. _____
2. _____
3. _____
4. _____
5. _____
6. _____
7. _____
8. _____
9. _____
10. _____
11. _____

Use the diagram to **circle** the areas of the body where **pressure ulcers** are likely to develop on a bedridden patient:

CLINICAL SITUATION   An 88-year-old female client has been admitted to the hospital with a fractured left elbow. She is malnourished and weighs only 90 lbs. She is currently confused and a sitter has been assigned at her bedside. The family reports that the client eats less than 50% of her meals and has difficulty walking. The client is anorexic and her skin is soft and thin. She is incontinent of urine.

Pertinent Terminology	Definition
Pressure Ulcer	
Necrosis	
Ischemia	
Reactive Hyperemia	
Blanching	
Slough	
Eschar	
Tunneling	
Debridement	
Excoriation	

BRADEN SCALE FOR PREDICTING PRESSURE SORE RISK

Go online and access the Braden Scale at *http://www.bradenscale.com/images/bradenscale.pdf*. **Select the number** on the scale that best applies to the client's risk for development of pressure ulcers (the **lower the number,** the greater is the risk for the development of pressure ulcers).

- After 2 days of taking care of the client, the nurse made the following documentation on the client's medical record: "Reddened, open, dry circular area on sacrum, approximately 2.5 cm × 2.5 cm. Dr. Stanley notified."
- Use the documentation to check off (✓) the **"stage"** of the client's pressure ulcer from the following **Pressure Ulcer Stages:**

Suspected Deep Tissue Injury	Stage I
☐ Purple or maroon discolored area; intact skin or blood-filled blister.	☐ Nonblanchable redness of a localized area; intact skin.
Stage II	**Stage III**
☐ Partial-thickness dermis loss. Pink wound bed without slough. May present as an intact or open serum-filled blister.	☐ Full-thickness tissue loss; subcutaneous fat may be visible, but bone, tendon, or muscle are not exposed. Slough, tunneling, and undermining may be present.
Stage IV	**Unstageable**
☐ Full-thickness tissue loss with exposed bone, tendon, or muscle. Slough and eschar may be present on some parts of the wound bed. Tunneling and undermining are often present.	☐ Full-thickness tissue loss in which the base of the ulcer is covered by slough or eschar.

Source: National Pressure Ulcer Advisory Board at *www.npuap.org*.

Collaborative Learning Activity: With a partner, **write in** the **"stage"** of the pressure ulcer for each of the following clinical situations using the **Pressure Ulcer Stages:**

Clinical Situation	Pressure Ulcer Stage
A male client was brought to the hospital. He has an open wound on his left heel that is 2 inches wide and 0.5 inches deep. It has a foul odor and the heel bone is exposed.	
The nurse measures an irregular open wound on the right hip. The subcutaneous tissue is visible.	

APPLYING CRITICAL THINKING SKILLS TO TEST QUESTIONS

INSTRUCTIONS: Circle the one best answer for each test question. Write your rationale for selecting the answer. To enhance your learning and test-taking skills, discuss your answer and rationale with a partner. The answer and the rationale can be found on the back of this page.

1. The nurse is taking care of a client who has a stage I pressure ulcer on the sacrum. In delegating the care of the client, it is most important for the nurse to:
   a. instruct the nursing assistant to turn the client every 2 hours.
   b. ask the nursing assistant to massage the client's sacrum.
   c. review how to assess the client's sacrum with the nursing assistant.
   d. inform the nursing assistant of the client's pressure ulcer.

   Rationale for your selection: _____
   _____
   _____
   _____
   _____
   _____

2. While reading the admission notes of a client, the nurse notes that the physician has identified eschar on the left heel. Which of the following assessments is most significant of this finding?
   a. A black scab-like area on the left heel.
   b. A bruised area on the left heel.
   c. A stage III pressure ulcer on the left heel.
   d. A stage IV pressure ulcer on the left heel.

   Rationale for your selection: _____
   _____
   _____
   _____
   _____
   _____

3. On turning a client to the lateral position, the nurse notes a reddened area on the right hip. Further assessment reveals intact skin with blanching at the site. Which of the following is the most appropriate nursing intervention?
   a. Notify the physician.
   b. Document the findings.
   c. Apply a dry sterile dressing.
   d. Document the presence of a stage I pressure ulcer.

   Rationale for your selection: _____
   _____
   _____
   _____
   _____
   _____

ANSWER KEY FOR
APPLYING CRITICAL THINKING SKILLS TO TEST QUESTIONS

HELPFUL HINTS: Read all test questions carefully. Identify key words in the question that will guide you in answering the question. In these test questions the **key words** to consider are **"most important," "most significant,"** and **"most appropriate."** Compare your rationale with the one in the test question.

1. The nurse is taking care of a client who has a stage I pressure ulcer on the sacrum. In delegating the care of the client, it is most important for the nurse to:
   a. instruct the nursing assistant to turn the client every 2 hours.
   b. ask the nursing assistant to massage the client's sacrum.
   c. review how to assess the client's sacrum with the nursing assistant.
   d. inform the nursing assistant of the client's pressure ulcer.

   Rationale: The answer is (a). Instructing the nursing assistant to carry out an intervention that would assist in preventing further skin breakdown is most important. Option (b) could cause more tissue damage; option (c) is not appropriate for a nursing assistant to assess; and option (d) is not client-centered and does not provide a specific intervention to assist the client.

2. While reading the admission notes of a client, the nurse notes that the physician has identified eschar on the left heel. Which of the following assessments is most significant of this finding?
   a. A black scab-like area on the left heel.
   b. A bruised area on the left heel.
   c. A stage III pressure ulcer on the left heel.
   d. A stage IV pressure ulcer on the left heel.

   Rationale: The answer is (a), which describes the appearance of eschar. Eschar must be debrided to "stage" the pressure ulcer. Options (b), (c), and (d) do not describe the finding.

3. On turning a client to the lateral position, the nurse notes a reddened area on the right hip. Further assessment reveals intact skin with blanching at the site. Which of the following is the most appropriate nursing intervention?
   a. Notify the physician.
   b. Document the findings.
   c. Apply a dry sterile dressing.
   d. Document the presence of a stage I pressure ulcer.

   Rationale: The answer is (b). A reddened area with intact skin and blanching indicates circulation to the site. Options (a) and (c) are not necessary at this time. For option (d), the findings do not support the definition of a stage I pressure ulcer.

1-12 COMMUNICATION

List essential **therapeutic communication techniques** used in a helping relationship:

- _____
- _____
- _____
- _____
- _____

- _____
- _____
- _____
- _____
- _____

Identify **nontherapeutic responses** that block the development of therapeutic communication:

- _____
- _____
- _____
- _____
- _____
- _____

Use the diagrams to identify the factors that influence communication.

CLINICAL SITUATION Casey, a student nurse, is in the clinical facility for the first time. She is assigned to a 70-year-old female client who was admitted with a fracture of the right hip. The client had her own business for 30 years but is now retired. She remains active in her community. The staff tells the student nurse that the client is a very cranky woman. As soon as Casey walks into the room she hears, "Well, it is about time! If I had to wait any longer I probably would starve to death." Casey responds softly, "I just started my shift."

Pertinent Terminology	Definition
Therapeutic Relationship Orientation Phase	_____ _____ _____
Working Phase	_____ _____ _____
Termination Phase	_____ _____
Paralanguage	_____ _____
Communication	_____ _____

Use the clinical situation to identify **three factors** that would initially affect the development of a therapeutic relationship with the client:

_____   _____   _____

Casey's response to the client is an example of _____
Casey may have addressed the client's statements by saying: _____
_____

Identify the **therapeutic communication technique** used by Casey in the statement and provide a **rationale** as to why this statement is more appropriate:

Therapeutic Technique	Rationale

Collaborative Learning Activity: With a partner, use the following clinical situations to select the appropriate communication technique or response being used:

Paraphrasing   False reassurance   Summarizing

Open-ended question   Clarification   Advising

1. **Nurse:** "Good morning Mr. S, I heard you had a lot of pain last night. Could you describe the type of pain you had?"

_____

2. **Family Member:** "The doctor just told me that my husband suffered a severe heart attack!"

   Nurse: "I'm sorry, but don't worry, I'm sure everything will be fine."

_____

3. **Client:** "I'm just so sick all the time. I just can't do anything by myself anymore. I feel so helpless!"

   Nurse: "It is hard for you to be so dependent and not feel like you are in control. You sound pretty tired of it all."

_____

4. **Client:** "Nurse, I need to know more information on the pill you gave me this morning."

   Nurse: "Mr. G, I gave you several pills this morning. Which one would you like to know more about?"

_____

APPLYING CRITICAL THINKING SKILLS TO TEST QUESTIONS

INSTRUCTIONS: Circle the one best answer for each test question. Write your rationale for selecting the answer. To enhance your learning and test-taking skills, discuss your answer and rationale with a partner. The answer and the rationale can be found on the back of this page.

1. The following conversation takes place at the client's bedside:
   Nurse: "Good morning Mr. J, I am your nurse for today. Did you sleep well?"
   Client: "I am not sure."
   Nurse: "You are not sure?"
   Which of the following statements is most accurate of this conversation? The nurse:
   a. should ask a question to validate the client's confusion.
   b. used an appropriate follow-up communication technique.
   c. should look at the chart to see how the client slept.
   d. was inappropriate in asking the second question.

   Rationale for your selection: _____
   _____
   _____
   _____
   _____
   _____

2. The nurse walks into a client's room and sees the postsurgical client holding his abdomen and grimacing. The nurse states, "You look like you are in pain." The nurse's statement is:
   a. appropriate because it states what the nurse is observing.
   b. appropriate because pain is expected after surgery.
   c. inappropriate because the nurse made a conclusion before validating.
   d. inappropriate because the nurse should wait for the client to speak first.

   Rationale for your selection: _____
   _____
   _____
   _____
   _____
   _____

3. The following conversation takes place at the client's bedside:
   Nurse: "Mr. T, I will be teaching you how to change your surgical dressing."
   Client: "I would prefer that you wait until my wife gets here. She takes care of everything."
   Nurse: "You shouldn't depend on your wife. I'll show you first and then you can teach your wife."
   The nurse's last statement is:
   a. advising the client.
   b. appropriate because it encourages self-care.
   c. having the client reinforce what will be taught.
   d. inappropriate because the nurse should have called the wife first.

   Rationale for your selection: _____
   _____
   _____
   _____
   _____
   _____

ANSWER KEY FOR
APPLYING CRITICAL THINKING SKILLS TO TEST QUESTIONS

HELPFUL HINTS: Read all test questions carefully. Identify key words in the question that will guide you in answering the question. In these test questions the **key words** to consider are **"most accurate"** and **"most important."** Compare your rationale with the one in the test question.

1. The following conversation takes place at the client's bedside:
   Nurse: "Good morning Mr. J, I am your nurse for today. Did you sleep well?"
   Client: "I am not sure."
   Nurse: "You are not sure?"
   Which of the following statements is most accurate of this conversation? The nurse:
   a. should ask a question to validate the client's confusion.
   b. used an appropriate follow-up communication technique.
   c. should look at the chart to see how the client slept.
   d. was inappropriate in asking the second question.

   Rationale: The answer is (b). The nurse used a reflective (paraphrase) technique to solicit more information from the client. Options (a), (c), and (d) do not solicit more information.

2. The nurse walks into a client's room and sees the postsurgical client holding his abdomen and grimacing. The nurse states, "You look like you are in pain." The nurse's statement is:
   a. appropriate because it states what the nurse is observing.
   b. appropriate because pain is expected after surgery.
   c. inappropriate because the nurse made a conclusion before validating.
   d. inappropriate because the nurse should wait for the client to speak first.

   Rationale: The answer is (a). The nurse is stating an objective observation. This allows the client to clarify or validate the observation. Options (b), (c), and (d) are not appropriate therapeutic communication techniques that facilitate client communication.

3. The following conversation takes place at the client's bedside:
   Nurse: "Mr. T, I will be teaching you how to change your surgical dressing."
   Client: "I would prefer that you wait until my wife gets here. She takes care of everything."
   Nurse: "You shouldn't depend on your wife. I'll show you first and then you can teach your wife."
   The nurse's last statement is:
   a. advising the client.
   b. appropriate because it encourages self-care.
   c. having the client reinforce what will be taught.
   d. inappropriate because the nurse should have called the wife first.

   Rationale: The answer is (a). The nurse's comment reflects how the nurse feels about the client's decision and does not demonstrate sensitivity to the client. This can cause a block in communication. Options (b), (c), and (d) do not take into consideration the importance of the client's personal needs and social structure.

1-13 INTRODUCTION TO THE ASSESSMENT PROCESS

List the **methods** available to the nurse for the **collection of patient data:**

1. _____
2. _____
3. _____
4. _____

List the parts of the patient's medical record that assist the nurse in the collection of patient data:

1. _____
2. _____
3. _____
4. _____
5. _____
6. _____

Draw a line to connect the **Objective Data.**

- Subjective
- "I have a headache."
- Gold-colored chain
- States nauseated
- Resp. 22 regular
- WBC is 5000/mm³
- Objective

CLINICAL SITUATION   Mrs. C has been admitted to the hospital for the birth of her baby. Her husband is by her side. You observe that she is very pleasant but cries out with each contraction. She tells you, "I feel a lot of pressure in my back." Her medical record indicates that she is 26 years old and that she has a 6-year-old son.

Pertinent Terminology	Definition
Assessment	
Subjective Data	
Objective Data	
Clustering Data	
Validation of Data	
Primary Source	
Secondary Source	

Use the clinical situation to identify the following information:

List the objective data:	Source (Primary/Secondary)
1.	
2.	
3.	
4.	
List the subjective data:	
1.	

Collaborative Learning Activity: With a partner, use the box to identify subjective and objective data from the clinical situations:

Mrs. T has been admitted with depression. She answers questions softly with a "yes" or "no" response. She wants her door closed and her room dark. She refuses visitors and eats only 10% of her meals. You notice that she cries regularly and sleeps a lot. She bites her nails frequently.	**Objective Data** **Subjective Data**
Mr. P had surgery 1 day ago. He tells you that he has been very independent all his life and hates being sick. He has refused his pain medication all morning. You notice that he refuses to get out of bed, he moans quietly every now and then, he is sweaty, and his hands are clenched tightly. His surgical dressing is clean and he says everything is fine when you ask him a question.	**Objective Data** **Subjective Data**
Mr. K informs the certified nursing assistant that he is nauseated. He has refused his lunch. You go in to check him and you notice 100 mL of clear yellow emesis. He tells you that he vomited. His wife is at his bedside.	**Objective Data** **Subjective Data**

1-14 BASIC PHYSICAL ASSESSMENT

List the **four methods of examination** used in the performance of a physical assessment:

1. _____
2. _____
3. _____
4. _____

Write in the most appropriate **method(s) of examination** for each of the following:

- Oral mucous membranes
  _____

- Peripheral pulses
  _____

- Arterial blood pressure
  _____

- Lung sounds
  _____

- Lower extremity edema
  _____

- Apical pulse
  _____

- Distended abdomen
  _____

CLINICAL SITUATION   Carrie is a nursing student assigned to Ms. W. Ms. W, 18 years old, came to the emergency department with complaints of right lower abdominal pain. She was admitted and had an appendectomy the day of admission. She is 1 day postop and will be going home this afternoon. Carrie performs a **body systems assessment** and documents the following notes on her clinical worksheet:

Neuro: Alert and oriented ×4. **Cardiovascular:** Radial pulse, regular and bounding. **Skin:** Warm and dry, pallor present, turgor elastic. **Respirations:** Regular, clear. **Gastrointestinal:** Bowel sounds present in all four quadrants. RLQ abdominal dressing clean, complains of tenderness with light palpation. **Genitourinary:** States voiding without difficulty. **Musculoskeletal:** Ambulates with a steady gait. **Psychosocial:** Cheerful.

Pertinent Terminology	Definition
Inspection	_____
Palpation	_____
Percussion	_____
	_____
	_____
Auscultation	_____
Chief Complaint	_____
Review of Systems	_____

Use the Body Systems Assessment Notes from the clinical situation to **identify the method of examination** used by Carrie in performing the body systems assessment:

Body Systems Assessment Notes	Method(s) of Examination
Neuro: Alert and oriented ×4	
Cardiovascular: Radial pulse regular and bounding	
Skin: Warm and dry, pallor, turgor elastic	
Respirations: Regular, clear	
Gastrointestinal: Bowel sounds present in all four quadrants. Right lower quadrant abdominal dressing clean; complains of tenderness with light palpation	
Genitourinary: States voiding without difficulty	
Musculoskeletal: Ambulates with a steady gait	
Psychosocial: Cheerful	

Collaborative Learning Activity: With a partner, use the following Assessment Notes to identify (1) the body system being assessed, and (2) the method of examination used:

Assessment Notes	Body System Method(s) of Examination
States it is 1945, does not know where he is; knows first name; hand grip strength unequal: right hand grip stronger than left	
Voided 50 mL of amber fluid; abdomen distended	
Warm, moist; pallor with erythema on sacral area; edema 1+ on bilateral lower extremities	
Absent bowel sounds in lower and upper right quadrants, hyperactive on upper and lower left quadrants; having small amounts of liquid dark brown stools	
Wheezes audible on inspiration, coughing, expectorating thick yellowish phlegm	
Apical pulse 116, rapid, irregular; radial pulse 98, rapid, thready, irregular	
Passive range of motion to right hand. Unable to extend and flex fingers	
Left facial drooping; left arm and leg flaccid	

APPLYING CRITICAL THINKING SKILLS TO TEST QUESTIONS

INSTRUCTIONS: Circle the one best answer for each test question. Write your rationale for selecting the answer. To enhance your learning and test-taking skills, discuss your answer and rationale with a partner. The answer and the rationale can be found on the back of this page.

1. The nurse is preparing to assess the neurologic status of an adult client who had a hip fracture 5 days ago and was reported to have been confused during the previous shift. Which statement will provide the nurse with the most appropriate information?
   a. "Can you tell me today's date?"
   b. "Do you know that you are in the hospital?"
   c. "When did you have hip surgery?"
   d. "Tell me where you are right now."

   Rationale for your selection: _____
   _____
   _____
   _____
   _____
   _____

2. The nurse is informed that a newly admitted client is complaining of itching and has a rash all over the body. The most appropriate nursing intervention initially is to:
   a. inform the physician of the objective and subjective complaints.
   b. inspect the client and describe the rash.
   c. ask the client to try not to scratch the areas.
   d. check the medication record for antiitch medication.

   Rationale for your selection: _____
   _____
   _____
   _____
   _____
   _____

3. The nurse is assigned to a client who was admitted for a blood clot in the right leg. Which of the following describes the appropriate assessment technique initially?
   a. Inspection of the right leg.
   b. Light palpation of the right leg.
   c. Inspection followed by deep palpation of edematous areas.
   d. Light palpation followed by inspection of any reddened areas.

   Rationale for your selection: _____
   _____
   _____
   _____
   _____
   _____

ANSWER KEY FOR
APPLYING CRITICAL THINKING SKILLS TO TEST QUESTIONS

HELPFUL HINTS: Read all test questions carefully. Identify key words in the question that will guide you in answering the question. In these test questions the **key words** to consider are **"most appropriate"** and **"initially."** Compare your rationale with the one in the test question.

1. The nurse is preparing to assess the neurologic status of an adult client who had a hip fracture 5 days ago and was reported to have been confused during the previous shift. Which statement will provide the nurse with the most appropriate information?
   a. "Can you tell me today's date?"
   b. "Do you know that you are in the hospital?"
   c. "When did you have hip surgery?"
   d. "Tell me where you are right now."

   Rationale: The answer is (d). Eliciting orientation to place is part of assessing client orientation. Options (a) and (b) encourage a "yes" or "no" response, and option (c) may not give accurate data if the client does not remember the date.

2. The nurse is informed that a newly admitted client is complaining of itching and has a rash all over the body. The most appropriate nursing intervention initially is to:
   a. inform the physician of the objective and subjective complaints.
   b. inspect the client and describe the rash.
   c. ask the client to try not to scratch the areas.
   d. check the medication record for antiitch medication.

   Rationale: The answer is (b). It is most appropriate for the nurse to initially gather data by using the assessment skill of inspection and then to further describe the observations. Options (a), (c), and (d) are follow-up nursing interventions.

3. The nurse is assigned to a client who was admitted for a blood clot in the right leg. Which of the following describes the appropriate assessment technique initially?
   a. Inspection of the right leg.
   b. Light palpation of the right leg.
   c. Inspection followed by deep palpation of edematous areas.
   d. Light palpation followed by inspection of any reddened areas.

   Rationale: The answer is (a). Inspection is the initial step in the assessment process that provides information on color, size, shape, and movement of the extremity. Options (b) and (d) are not appropriate initially, and option (c) should not be done in this situation.

1-15 USING SBAR TO REPORT PATIENT STATUS

List the most common methods nurses use to **report patient status** during the shift and from shift to shift:

1. _____

2. _____

3. _____

Place an "X" in the box(es) that best describe(s) the information that should be included in a **handoff report.** The handoff report should:

☐ Provide basic information such as room number, date of admission, and medical diagnosis.
☐ Provide specific information regarding the client's needs and plan of care.
☐ Provide information on significant changes in the client's condition.
☐ Provide information on follow-up client care.
☐ Provide information on clients transferred or discharged from the unit.

CLINICAL SITUATION

0700 Handoff Report

S Mr. J in room 461 is a 76-year-old man. He was admitted last night with sepsis.

B He has an IV of 0.9% normal saline infusing at 75 mL/hr. He has been NPO but is allowed sips of water. His 0200 temp was 99.2°F.

A He has been restless since he woke up at 0500, and he is not oriented to time and place. He says that it is 2005 and that he is at home. The 0600 temperature was 100.6°F, and his blood pressure is 146/94. I gave him acetaminophen at 0615. His output for the shift was 150 mL total.

R I am concerned about his temperature and output; I left a message with his doctor at 0630. It is important to monitor his temperature this morning and notify his physician about his confusion and his output when he calls back.

Pertinent Terminology	Definition
Handoff Report	
Electronic Health Record (EHR)	
Electronic Medical Record (EMR) Worksheet	
Reporting	
SBAR	

Use the **0700 Handoff Report** to identify the <u>**immediate follow-up**</u> patient care.

Identify the Immediate Follow-up Care	Rationale
Assess confusion, restlessness	Maintain patient safety. Identify need for frequent monitoring, assessment, use of side rails, etc.
Take current vital signs	Assess current VS; establish baseline and compare with previous VS.
Assess output and IV site/infusion	Ensure IV infusion is on time. Assess urine color, odor, and amount.
Perform a body systems assessment	Gather baseline data.
Check results of admission laboratory work	Gather data; follow-up on abnormal results.
Check Code status	Sepsis is a life-threatening condition. It is important to provide nursing that minimizes further complications, promotes safe practices, focuses on patient-centered care, and maintains patient comfort.

Collaborative Learning Activity: With a partner, read the **0700-1500 Recorded Assessment Notes** below to gather information regarding the care given to Mr. J. during the shift.

	Recorded Assessment Notes
0745	Physician called notified of confusion and restlessness.
0900	AM care provided. Side rails up.
1000	VS 101.2 –98–28 138/90 SpO$_2$ 92%
1200	VS 102.6 – 100 –28 130/88 SpO$_2$ 90% Oxygen started via nasal cannula at 3 L/min. Acetaminophen administered for fever greater than 101.4.
1400	VS 102 –100 –28 128/88 SpO$_2$ 90% Difficult to assess pain level. Oxygen at 3 L/min. Skin flushed, warm, Crackles on ® lower lung base, IV patent. Confused, lethargic. Incontinent of urine. Will be transferred to critical care when bed available.

Use the SBAR format below to write the **handoff report that will be given at 1500.**

S	Mr. J in room 461 is a 76-year-old man. He is diagnosed with sepsis.
B	He has been confused all shift and has had a fever since the night shift. He received acetaminophen at 1200 for a fever of 102.6°F.
A	He is awake, lethargic, and confused to time and place. 1400 vital signs are: 102–100–28 128/88 SpO$_2$ 90%. Difficult to assess pain level. Skin is warm and flushed. Crackles audible on the ® lower lung base. Oxygen at 3 L/min.
R	He will be transferred to critical care when a bed is available. Until he is transferred, I recommend that his VS be monitored q15min and report changes in orientation.

1-16 DOCUMENTATION

List the various documentation (charting) formats used in the clinical settings:

1. _____
2. _____
3. _____
4. _____
5. _____
6. _____

Circle the statements that are **true.**

The patient's medical record is a communication tool.

The RN is legally responsible for the documentation made by student nurses.

Charting entries should be concise.

Flow sheets are not part of the client's chart.

Pertinent Terminology	Definition
APIE Charting	_____
Charting by Exception	_____
Clinical Pathway	_____
Electronic Charting Narrative Charting	_____
Flow Sheets Focus Charting	_____
POMR Charting	_____
SOAP Charting	_____

Example #1 Nonelectronic (paper) documentation

Nurses' Notes

Time	
0800	Alert, oriented ×4. States pain level 5 out of 10, using PCA. Lung sounds clear, unlabored using incentive spirometer. Skin warm, dry. NG to suction draining light brown fluid. BS absent ×4 quads. Abd dressing with 2 cm × 2 cm pinkish drainage._____M. Molly RN
0900	Foley discontinued as ordered._____ M. Molly RN

Charting format: _____

Example #2

```
┌──────────────────────────────────────────────────────────────────┐ _ □ X
│                                                                    │
│  Name: Joe Smith    Age: 56    Sex: Male      Code status: Full    Allergies: NKDA │
│  ID # 125673        BD: 10/30/xx   Rm: 205       J. Zerne M.D.      Dx: Pneumonia   │
│                                                                    │
│  Day/Time: Monday / 1500           MMaz RN                         │
│  **Respiratory Assessment**                                        │
│  Rate: 28     SpO₂ 94%    Sputum ◉    Color  Yellow ▾   Cough ◉    │
│  Pattern:  Regular ◯  Labored ◉   Shallow ◯   Deep ◯              │
│                                                                    │
│  **Lung Auscultation**                                             │
│                          ◯ Fine Crackles   ◉ Coarse Crackles      │
│                          ◯ Rhonchi         ◯ Wheeze               │
│                          ◯ Diminished      ◯ Absent               │
│                                                                    │
│                          Notes:                                    │
│                          Started on O₂ at 3L/min via NP.           │
│                          High Fowler's position.                   │
└──────────────────────────────────────────────────────────────────┘
```

1. Identify how the data entered guides the patient plan of care. _____
_____
_____

⚙️ **Collaborative Learning Activity:** With a partner, use the following **nonelectronic narrative notes** to identify charting mistake entries. List how these entries should be corrected.

Nonelectronic Narrative Notes	
Time	
0700	Patient sleeping. Resp. 20 regular, unlabored. Skin warm_____ M. Molly RN
0730	Awake, pain level 0. Patient up to bathroom MAEW. c/o dizziness on returning to bed. Pale, assisted back to bed. P 98, irregular. BP 90/60 no c/o pain. Side rails up ×4. _____ M. Molly RN
0830	Patient refused breakfast, c/o mild indegestion. Will check to see what medications are ordered _____ _____ M. Molly RN
0900	Had emesis of 100 mL stated, "Felt better" _____ M. Molly RN

Charting errors:

1. _____
   Correct by: _____

2. _____
   Correct by: _____

3. _____
   Correct by: _____

4. _____
   Correct by: _____

5. _____
   Correct by: _____

1-17 SELF-CONCEPT

List the **four components** of self-concept:

1. _____
2. _____
3. _____
4. _____

For each of the **self-concept** components, **identify two stressors** that affect and contribute to altering the component of:

➤ Identity (any two)
_____
_____
_____

➤ Body image (any two)
_____
_____

➤ Self-esteem (any two)
_____
_____
_____
_____

➤ Role performance (any two)
_____
_____
_____

CLINICAL SITUATION A female client was diagnosed with breast cancer 2 weeks ago and recently had a left mastectomy. She is 32 years old and is married with a 5-year-old daughter. She is very anxious after the surgery and wonders how her husband will react to her. She tells the nurse, "I am so young to have this done." She begins to cry and says that she loves being a mom but doesn't think she can have another child because she would not be able to nurse and care for the baby as she would like to. She is scheduled to begin chemotherapy treatments in 1 week.

Pertinent Terminology	Definition
Self-Concept	
Identity	
Body Image	
Self-Esteem	
Role Performance	

Reread the clinical situation and cluster the **objective data** and **subjective data** that relate to the **self-concept** component that is marked with an **"X":**

☐ Identity ☒ Body image ☐ Self-esteem ☐ Role performance	➡	**Objective data:**
	➡	**Subjective data:**
☐ Identity ☐ Body image ☐ Self-esteem ☒ Role performance	➡	**Objective data:**
	➡	**Subjective data:**

Collaborative Learning Activity: With a partner, use the following clinical situation to cluster the objective data and the subjective data related to the **self-concept** component that is marked with an **"X."**

CLINICAL SITUATION A male client had a heart attack 2 months ago and has lost his job. When he comes to the clinic his facial expression is tense and he speaks in a hostile voice. During the last visit, he stated: "I can't just sit here, I am the breadwinner of my family." "I'm useless since I had the heart attack!"

☒ Identity ☐ Body image ☐ Self-esteem ☐ Role performance	➡	**Objective data:**
	➡	**Subjective data:**
☐ Identity ☐ Body image ☒ Self-esteem ☐ Role performance	➡	**Objective data:**
	➡	**Subjective data:**

1-18 CULTURAL ASPECTS OF NURSING

List the **six cultural variables** that influence nursing care:

1. _____

2. _____

3. _____

4. _____

5. _____

6. _____

List **two examples** for each of the following:

Communication

_____

_____

Social organizations

_____

_____

Environmental control

_____

_____

Biological variations

_____

_____

_____

CLINICAL SITUATION   Wendy RN, the home health nurse, visits a 62-year-old Hispanic woman who has had diabetes mellitus (DM) for 20 years and currently has a sore on her left foot. The client has missed two of her doctor's appointments and has been soaking her foot in warm salt water every night. The client speaks English but does not like to call the clinic or question the nurse because she does not want to bother anyone. She enjoys cooking and eating Mexican food. During the home visit Wendy noticed several religious artifacts and many pictures of the client's children and grandchildren on the wall.

Pertinent Terminology	Definition
Culture	
Culture Assessment	
Cultural Sensitivity	
Cultural Imposition	
Assimilation	
Ethnocentrism	

1 Knowledge Application

Use the clinical situation to **identify** the **cultural data** that relate to the **culture variables** listed below:

Culture Variables	Cultural Data
Communication	
Space	
Time	
Social organization	
Environmental control	
Biological variation	

Collaborative Learning Activity: With a partner, use the following clinical situations to (1) underline the pertinent cultural data and (2) identify the possible implications for health care delivery:

Clinical Situation	Health Care Delivery Implication(s)
A Filipino woman is very quiet. She rarely complains and the nurses comment on how she does not maintain eye contact when the nurse is speaking.	
A client of Chinese ancestry is 80 years old and requires constant care. She lives with one of her daughters and all the adult family members are involved in caring for her at night.	
Mrs. W has had a miscarriage. She hemorrhaged and her blood count is very low. The physician has recommended a blood transfusion, but Mrs. W refuses because of her religious beliefs.	
An African American woman comes to the outpatient clinic for blood pressure checks. She tells the nurse that her youngest daughter is about to be married. She is concerned because her other daughter has sickle cell anemia.	
A male client had major surgery yesterday. He does not want to get out of bed and has refused all his pain medication. The nurse knows that he is in pain but wants to respect his wishes.	

APPLYING CRITICAL THINKING SKILLS TO TEST QUESTIONS

INSTRUCTIONS: Circle the one best answer for each test question. Write your rationale for selecting the answer. To enhance your learning and test-taking skills, discuss your answer and rationale with a partner. The answer and the rationale can be found on the back of this page.

1. The nurse is preparing to discuss with the alert elderly Hispanic female client the bronchoscopy procedure scheduled the next day. The client tells the nurse that she wants to wait until her family arrives later. Which nursing action is most appropriate?
   a. Provide the information to the client and answer the family's questions later.
   b. Give the client the bronchoscopy procedure information in Spanish.
   c. Tell the client to call you when her family arrives.
   d. Inform the physician.

   Rationale for your selection: _____
   _____
   _____
   _____
   _____
   _____

2. The nurse is taking care of a client who is scheduled for surgery today. The client asks the nurse to read a passage from the Bible to help her prepare herself for surgery. It is most appropriate for the nurse to:
   a. read the Bible passage.
   b. ask if someone on staff is the same religion as the client.
   c. kindly tell the client that nurses cannot get involved in religious issues.
   d. inquire whether the client would prefer that a religious person be called.

   Rationale for your selection: _____
   _____
   _____
   _____
   _____
   _____

3. The nurse is assigned to a client who believes that wearing a copper bracelet will relieve arthritic pain. In providing care for the client, it is most important for the nurse to:
   a. encourage the client to use antiinflammatory medication.
   b. inform the client that copper bracelets have no proven medical value.
   c. address the pathophysiologic mechanisms associated with arthritis with the client.
   d. respect the beliefs associated with the copper bracelet by the client.

   Rationale for your selection: _____
   _____
   _____
   _____
   _____
   _____

ANSWER KEY FOR
APPLYING CRITICAL THINKING SKILLS TO TEST QUESTIONS

HELPFUL HINTS: Read all test questions carefully. Identify key words in the question that will guide you in answering the question. In these test questions the **key words** to consider are **"most appropriate"** and **"most important."** Compare your rationale with the one in the test question.

1. The nurse is preparing to discuss with the alert elderly Hispanic female client the bronchoscopy procedure scheduled the next day. The client tells the nurse that she wants to wait until her family arrives later. Which nursing action is most appropriate?
   a. Provide the information to the client and answer the family's questions later.
   b. Give the client the bronchoscopy procedure information in Spanish.
   (c.) Tell the client to call you when her family arrives.
   d. Inform the physician.

   Rationale: The answer is (c). The family is an important social organization in many cultures. Being available when the family arrives is manifesting respect for the client's wishes and cultural sensitivity. Options (a) and (d) do not address cultural sensitivity. Although option (b) demonstrates cultural sensitivity, this initial action assumes the client wants the information in Spanish. It would be preferable to ask the client if she would like the information in English or Spanish.

2. The nurse is taking care of a client who is scheduled for surgery today. The client asks the nurse to read a passage from the Bible to help her prepare herself for surgery. It is most appropriate for the nurse to:
   (a.) read the Bible passage.
   b. ask if someone on staff is the same religion as the client.
   c. kindly tell the client that nurses cannot get involved in religious issues.
   d. inquire whether the client would prefer that a religious person be called.

   Rationale: The answer is (a). Recognizing the spiritual needs of a client is viewing the client as a whole person, with spiritual and physical needs. Options (b), (c), and (d) defer the needs of the patient to someone else.

3. The nurse is assigned to a client who believes that wearing a copper bracelet will relieve arthritic pain. In providing care for the client, it is most important for the nurse to:
   a. encourage the client to use antiinflammatory medication.
   b. inform the client that copper bracelets have no proven medical value.
   c. address the pathophysiologic mechanisms associated with arthritis with the client.
   (d.) respect the beliefs associated with the copper bracelet by the client.

   Rationale: The answer is (d). Cultural beliefs play an important role in the healing process. This cultural belief does not interfere with the client's well-being. Options (a), (b), and (c) tend to minimize the client's belief.

1-19 DEVELOPING CULTURALLY COMPETENT CARE

List **factors** that **increase cultural awareness**:

1. _____

_____

2. _____

_____

The **Health Care Culture Compass** identifies relevant human experiences and cultural needs encountered in the health care setting. Nurses need to develop an awareness of their own cultural beliefs and values in order to provide culturally competent care.

(Other human experiences and cultural needs such as privacy, family role, etc., may be substituted on the health care culture compass.)

CLINICAL SITUATION   The nurse is assigned to Mrs. C, a 45-year-old female patient, who was in a motor vehicle accident. The medical history indicates that Mrs. C is from another country, and she was traveling alone on vacation. She has terminal lung cancer. The patient is conscious but in very critical condition. Per her request, a do-not-resuscitate (DNR) order is written. Her only son will arrive in 3 days.

Pertinent Terminology	Definition
Cultural Awareness	_____
	_____
	_____
Cultural Competence	_____
	_____
Culturally Competent Care	_____
Patient-Centered Care	_____
	_____
	_____

Use the health care compass to:

(1) Think about **your own cultural views and beliefs** related to the cultural area identified by the arrow. Then, fill in the answer below.

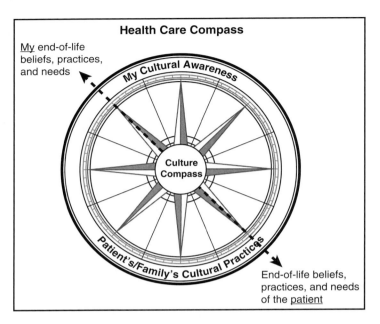

Your own end-of-life beliefs:

• Spiritual/religious beliefs and practices related to end-of-life care: _____
_____

Collaborative Learning Activity: With a partner, use the clinical situation of Mrs. C to:

• Identify questions that provide the nurse with **knowledge** of Mrs. C's end-of-life cultural beliefs and needs.
_____
_____
_____
_____

• Identify nursing interventions that reflect **patient-centered culturally competent care.**
_____
_____
_____
_____

• As Mrs. C is becoming progressively weaker, she whispers to the nurse that her greatest fear is "dying alone." Identify nursing interventions that would comfort Mrs. C during this time.
_____
_____
_____
_____

1-20 INTRODUCTION TO FORMULATING A NURSING DIAGNOSIS

List the five steps of the nursing process:

1. _____
2. _____
3. _____
4. _____
5. _____

The **NANDA-I nursing diagnoses** are classified and formulated to address the client's health problems or needs, which can be:

1. _____
2. _____
3. _____
4. _____

Use the book to write the NANDA-I definition for the following nursing diagnoses.

Nursing Diagnosis	NANDA-I Definition
Ineffective breathing pattern -	_____
Impaired gas exchange -	_____
Acute pain -	_____
Risk for infection -	_____

CLINICAL SITUATION   The home health nurse makes the following observations and documents the assessment findings after visiting a 68-year-old male client: lives alone; his only son lives 60 miles away, visits monthly, and calls weekly. The client stays indoors all day. His vision is poor and he is not able to drive.

Pertinent Terminology	Definition
NANDA-I	_____
Nursing Process	_____
Assessment	_____
Nursing Diagnosis	_____
Defining Characteristics	_____
Planning	_____
Implementation	_____
Evaluation	_____
Related to Factors	_____

From the clinical situation, **check off (✓) the nursing diagnosis** most appropriate for the client (use a nursing diagnosis book to validate your selection):

Nursing diagnoses: ___ Ineffective coping
___ Risk for loneliness
___ Social isolation

List the <u>risk factors</u> or defining characteristics for the nursing diagnosis you selected:

_____   _____   _____

_____   _____

IP **Further documentation** by the home health nurse states: The client has lost 10 lbs since the last visit 2 weeks ago. He now demonstrates signs of being malnourished. He lives on a limited income. Needs the services of a nutritionist and a local community service that delivers meals to homebound individuals.

From the **further documentation data, check off (✓) the nursing diagnosis** most appropriate for the client:

Nursing diagnoses: ___ Social isolation
___ Deficient knowledge
___ Imbalanced nutrition: less than body requirements

List the **current pertinent defining characteristics** for the nursing diagnosis you selected:

_____   _____   _____

Collaborative Learning Activity: With a partner, review the following clinical situations and **identify** the **defining characteristics** that relate to the **nursing diagnosis** written next to each situation.

Clinical Situation	Defining Characteristics
The client has a stage II pressure ulcer on her right heel. She has been on bed rest and her right leg is elevated.	IMPAIRED SKIN INTEGRITY _____
The client has oral lesions in his mouth 1 week after receiving chemotherapy. He complains of pain and his mouth is red.	IMPAIRED ORAL MUCOUS MEMBRANES _____
The client is scheduled for surgery in the morning. She says that she is very scared because her grandmother died during surgery.	FEAR _____

1-21 FORMULATING A NURSING DIAGNOSIS

Identify the components that need to be included in the development of:

Health promotion nursing diagnosis:

1. _____

2. _____

Risk nursing diagnosis:

1. _____

2. _____

Problem-focused nursing diagnosis:

1. _____

2. _____

3. _____

Place an "X" in the box that identifies the common errors made in the development of the nursing diagnosis statement:

☐ Using the NANDA-I diagnostic categories to identify the nursing diagnosis

☐ Using the medical diagnosis in the formulation of the nursing diagnosis

☐ Clustering the subjective/objective data

☐ Using signs and symptoms to write the nursing diagnosis statement

☐ Stating the expected outcome and the diagnostic statement

☐ Using subjective and objective data to identify the nursing diagnosis

☐ Being specific in defining the etiology part of the statement

☐ Stating the medical diagnosis as the etiology

CLINICAL SITUATION   The client is to be scheduled for elective surgery. In preparation for the surgery, the office nurse takes the client's health history. The nurse documents that the client has recently been diagnosed with diabetes mellitus type 2 and was prescribed an antidiabetic pill to take every morning. The client tells the nurse that she stopped the "pill" 1 week ago because she was feeling better.

Pertinent Terminology	Definition
Problem-Focused Nursing Diagnosis	_____ _____
Risk Nursing Diagnosis	_____ _____ _____
Health Promotion Nursing Diagnosis	_____ _____
Risk Factors	_____ _____
Etiology	_____ _____
Data Cluster	_____ _____

Use **the clinical situation** to **cluster** the **subjective** and **objective data.**

Objective data: _____

Subjective data: _____

Use the data to complete a problem-focused nursing diagnosis for the client:

Deficient knowledge: _____
_____

Collaborative Learning Activity: With a partner, review the following clinical situations and (1) list the defining characteristics, (2) identify the error in the nursing diagnosis statement, and (3) write a correct nursing diagnosis.

CLINICAL SITUATION

Throughout the morning, the 66-year-old client has become progressively confused. He is restless and attempted to get out of bed. He says it is "1982." His laboratory diagnostic studies indicate that he has a decreased serum sodium level and is febrile. The nurse wrote the following nursing diagnosis:

Chronic confusion, related to electrolyte imbalance

Defining Characteristics
_____
_____

Error(s)
_____
_____
_____
_____
_____

Nursing Diagnosis
_____
_____
_____
_____
_____
_____

The client goes weekly to the outpatient clinic to have his blood pressure checked. He smokes one pack of cigarettes per day. His blood pressure is 146/88. His father died from heart disease at age 49, and his brother is recovering from a heart attack. The nurse writes the following nursing diagnosis:

Risk for heart attack related to smoking and family history of heart disease.

Related to Factors
_____
_____
_____
_____
_____

Error(s)
_____
_____
_____
_____
_____

Nursing Diagnosis
_____
_____
_____
_____
_____

APPLYING CRITICAL THINKING SKILLS TO TEST QUESTIONS

INSTRUCTIONS: Circle the one best answer for each test question. Write your rationale for selecting the answer. To enhance your learning and test-taking skills, discuss your answer and rationale with a partner. The answer and the rationale can be found on the back of this page.

1. The nurse clusters the client's objective and subjective signs and symptoms primarily to:
   a. identify the nursing diagnosis.
   b. correlate with the medical diagnosis.
   c. validate the subjective complaints.
   d. work with "risk for" diagnoses.

   Rationale for your selection:_____
   _____
   _____
   _____
   _____
   _____

2. The following nursing diagnosis is found on the patient's plan of care: Hip fracture related to fall. In evaluating the written nursing diagnosis, the nurse correctly concludes that the nursing diagnosis:
   a. is written inappropriately.
   b. should be a "risk for" nursing diagnosis.
   c. needs to be connected using "as evidenced by."
   d. needs the word "acute" before hip fracture.

   Rationale for your selection:_____
   _____
   _____
   _____
   _____
   _____

3. The nurse admits an elderly client with the medical diagnosis of dehydration. In developing the nursing diagnoses, it is most important for the nurse to:
   a. establish nursing diagnoses that are based on the medical diagnosis.
   b. focus on nursing diagnoses that affect fluid balance.
   c. gather data to support problem-focused nursing diagnoses.
   d. include problem-focused and "risk for" diagnoses.

   Rationale for your selection:_____
   _____
   _____
   _____
   _____
   _____

ANSWER KEY FOR
APPLYING CRITICAL THINKING SKILLS TO TEST QUESTIONS

HELPFUL HINTS: Read all test questions carefully. Identify key words in the question that will guide you in answering the question. In these test questions the **key words** to consider are **"primarily," "correctly concludes,"** and **"most important."** Compare your rationale with the one in the test question.

1. The nurse clusters the client's objective and subjective signs and symptoms primarily to:
   a. identify the nursing diagnosis.
   b. correlate with the medical diagnosis.
   c. validate the subjective complaints.
   d. work with "risk for" diagnoses.

   Rationale: The answer is (a). Clustering the data helps the nurse to identify the defining characteristic that led to the formulation of a nursing diagnosis. Options (b) and (c) do not apply, and option (d) addresses only "risk for" diagnoses.

2. The following nursing diagnosis is found on the patient's plan of care: Hip fracture related to fall. In evaluating the written nursing diagnosis, the nurse correctly concludes that the nursing diagnosis:
   a. is written inappropriately.
   b. should be a "risk for" nursing diagnosis.
   c. needs to be connected using "as evidenced by."
   d. needs the word "acute" before hip fracture.

   Rationale: The answer is (a). Hip fracture is a medical diagnosis. The nurse needs to identify the defining characteristics and then select the appropriate nursing diagnosis. Option (b) is not applicable because hip fracture is an actual client problem, and (c) and (d) do not apply to this example.

3. The nurse admits an elderly client with the medical diagnosis of dehydration. In developing the nursing diagnoses, it is most important for the nurse to:
   a. establish nursing diagnoses that are based on the medical diagnosis.
   b. focus on nursing diagnoses that affect fluid balance.
   c. gather data to support problem-focused nursing diagnoses.
   d. include problem-focused and "risk for" diagnoses.

   Rationale: The answer is (d). Nursing includes the development of problem-focused nursing diagnoses and any "risk for" diagnoses to provide total, safe care to the client. Option (a) is not correct, and options (b) and (c) do not include the monitoring of possible complications.

1-22 ASSESSMENT OF THE ELDERLY PATIENT

List the **interventions** that assist in communicating with an elderly patient who has hearing loss related to the aging process:

1. _____
2. _____
3. _____
4. _____
5. _____
6. _____

List the **interventions** that assist an elderly patient who has vision problems related to the aging process:

1. _____
2. _____
3. _____
4. _____
5. _____
6. _____

Mark an "**X**" in the appropriate column that identifies the effects of aging on the following:

	Decreased	Increased
Sensory perception	☐	☐
Visual acuity	☐	☐
Gag reflex	☐	☐
Skin tissue elasticity	☐	☐
Body temperature	☐	☐
Cardiac output	☐	☐
RBC production	☐	☐
Plasma viscosity	☐	☐
Lung capacity	☐	☐
Residual urine	☐	☐

CLINICAL SITUATION   The following information has been given to a group of students regarding the assessment of an elderly patient: Responds slowly but appropriately to all questions. Skin warm, dry, thin, and flaky. Skin turgor greater than 3 seconds. Capillary refill greater than 3 seconds. Respirations short and shallow, lung sounds with bilateral crackles. 50% intake, states food is very bland. BM this morning moderate amount formed hard stool. Bilateral lower extremities with +1 pitting edema. Toenails yellowish, thick. Vital signs: T 99°F, P 84, R 16, BP 160/80.

Pertinent Terminology	Definition
Arcus Senilis	_____
Edema	_____
Pitting Edema	_____
Kyphosis	_____
Presbycusis	_____
Presbyopia	_____
Turgor	_____

Use the information from the clinical situation to mark an **"X"** on the data that are representative of the normal effects of the aging process:

____   Responds slowly, but appropriately to all questions
____   Skin warm, dry, thin, and flaky
____   Skin turgor greater than 3 seconds; capillary refill greater than 3 seconds
____   Respirations short and shallow, lung sounds with bilateral crackles
____   50% intake, states food is very bland
____   BM this morning formed hard stool
____   Bilateral lower extremities with +1 pitting edema
____   Toenails yellowish, thick
____   Vital signs: T 99°F, P 84, R 16, BP 160/80

Collaborative Learning Activity: With a partner, use the information provided to (1) **underline** the assessment data that represent the **effects of the normal aging process** and (2) **select** the NANDA-I nursing diagnosis most appropriate for the situation:

Assessment Data	Nursing Diagnosis
Wife in to see patient, states that husband is confused this morning, does not know that he is in the hospital. Further patient assessment: PERRL, whitish ring noted around the margins of the iris, uses glasses. Mouth dry, wears upper dentures.	☐ Disturbed body image ☐ Impaired oral mucous membrane ☐ Acute confusion ☐ Impaired memory
Skin pale, translucent. Lower extremities thin, pedal pulses weak, palpable. States has loss of a small amount of urine when coughs. Shortness of breath, R 28, mouth breathing. Abdomen round, soft, non-tender. Temp. 96.8°F.	☐ Functional urinary incontinence ☐ Hypothermia ☐ Ineffective peripheral tissue perfusion ☐ Ineffective breathing pattern
Transfers independently out of bed, complained of dizziness when coming to a standing position, gait slow. Anterior-posterior diameter of chest increased. Soft diet, intake 70%.	☐ Impaired physical mobility ☐ Risk for injury ☐ Ineffective health maintenance ☐ Imbalanced nutrition: less than body requirements

1-23 CARING FOR THE SURGICAL PATIENT

List the **major** types of anesthesia:

1. _____

2. _____

3. _____

List the types of regional anesthesia:

1. _____

2. _____

3. _____

4. _____

5. _____

Identify in which of the perioperative phases (**preoperative, intraoperative, postoperative**) the following interventions would be started:

	Pre	Intra	Post
Use of incentive spirometer	☐	☐	☐
Coughing and deep breathing	☐	☐	☐
Splinting of surgical site	☐	☐	☐
Prepping surgical site	☐	☐	☐
Changing the surgical dressing	☐	☐	☐
Leg exercises	☐	☐	☐
Pain management	☐	☐	☐
Discharge instructions	☐	☐	☐

CLINICAL SITUATION A female patient is admitted for a total abdominal hysterectomy this morning. She is 52 years old and obese. Her medical history indicates that she stopped smoking 5 years ago. Both parents are deceased. Mother died at the age of 88 and father died from a heart attack at the age of 62. The patient's vital signs are T 97.8°F, P 76, R 18, BP 164/92, pain level 0. The following laboratory studies were done: CBC, PT, serum electrolytes of Na^+, K^+, serum FBG, BUN, and creatinine. The UA, chest x-ray report, and ECG report are available in the electronic health record.

Pertinent Terminology	Definition
General Anesthesia	
Regional Anesthesia	
Conscious Sedation	
Thrombophlebitis Atelectasis Paralytic Ileus	
PCA	
Sequential Stockings	

From the clinical situation, **list** the factors that increase the patient's risk for postoperative complications:

_____   _____

_____   _____

Collaborative Learning Activity: With a partner, use the follow-up clinical situation to (1) **identify** which medical order the nurse would do **first** and (2) list the **priority nursing interventions** the nurse would **independently** perform and provide a rationale for each intervention:

FOLLOW-UP CLINICAL SITUATION   The patient returns from the postanesthesia room sleepy but easily arousable. The postoperative orders include:

NPO, May have sips of water in the AM
IV: Dextrose 5/0.9% sodium chloride infuse at 100 mL/hr
Ambulate this evening
VS q30 min for first hour, then q1h ×2 hr, then q4h
Incentive spirometer q1h while awake
PCA with morphine sulfate set at 1 mg/6 min (per patient demand, not to exceed 30 mg/4 hr)
Antiembolic stockings and sequential stockings to legs continuously
Indwelling urinary catheter to gravity; remove in AM

First Medical Orders to Implement	Rationale
1.	
Priority Independent Nursing Interventions	**Rationale**
1.	
2.	
3.	
4.	
5.	
6.	
7.	

APPLYING CRITICAL THINKING SKILLS TO TEST QUESTIONS

INSTRUCTIONS: Circle the one best answer for each test question. Write your rationale for selecting the answer. To enhance your learning and test-taking skills, discuss your answer and rationale with a partner. The answer and the rationale can be found on the back of this page.

1. The client is transferred to the surgical unit from the postanesthesia room after having abdominal surgery. There is a J-P drainage device in place. Which of the following reported findings on transfer requires immediate follow-up?
   a. Abdominal dressing reinforced in the recovery room.
   b. R 14, P 86, BP 126/90, lethargic but responds to touch.
   c. Bowel sounds absent in all quadrants.
   d. J-P compressed with 10 mL reddish drainage.

   Rationale for your selection: _____
   _____
   _____
   _____
   _____
   _____

2. Which of the following client statements is correct in describing the appropriate use of the incentive spirometer?
   a. "I will first inhale then blow into the mouthpiece."
   b. "I will put the mouthpiece in my mouth and blow into it."
   c. "I will put the mouthpiece in my mouth and then inhale slowly."
   d. "I will put the mouthpiece in my mouth, inhale, and hold for 5 seconds."

   Rationale for your selection: _____
   _____
   _____
   _____
   _____
   _____

3. The nurse is preparing a client for emergency surgery. Before surgery, it is most important for the nurse to ensure that the:
   a. preop checklist is completed.
   b. preop medications are documented.
   c. lab results are in the medical record.
   d. surgical consent is signed.

   Rationale for your selection: _____
   _____
   _____
   _____
   _____
   _____

ANSWER KEY FOR
APPLYING CRITICAL THINKING SKILLS TO TEST QUESTIONS

HELPFUL HINTS: Read all test questions carefully. Identify key words in the question that will guide you in answering the question. In these test questions the **key words** to consider are **"immediate," "correct,"** and **"most important."** Compare your rationale with the one in the test question.

1. The client is transferred to the surgical unit from the postanesthesia room after having abdominal surgery. There is a J-P drainage device in place. Which of the following reported findings on transfer requires immediate follow-up?
    a. Abdominal dressing reinforced in the recovery room.
    b. R 14, P 86, BP 126/90, lethargic but responds to touch.
    c. Bowel sounds absent in all quadrants.
    d. J-P compressed with 10 mL reddish drainage.

    Rationale: The answer is (a). Reinforcement of the surgical dressing indicates excessive drainage; this should be carefully monitored. Option (b) indicates vital signs within normal limits, and options (c) and (d) are expected findings for a client who had abdominal surgery.

2. Which of the following client statements is correct in describing the appropriate use of the incentive spirometer?
    a. "I will first inhale then blow into the mouthpiece."
    b. "I will put the mouthpiece in my mouth and blow into it."
    c. "I will put the mouthpiece in my mouth and then inhale slowly."
    d. "I will put the mouthpiece in my mouth, inhale, and hold for 5 seconds."

    Rationale: The answer is (c). This describes the procedure appropriately. Options (a) and (b) do not describe the procedure correctly, and option (d) is partially correct but the client does not need to hold for 5 seconds.

3. The nurse is preparing a client for emergency surgery. Before surgery, it is most important for the nurse to ensure that the:
    a. preop checklist is completed.
    b. preop medications are documented.
    c. lab results are in the medical record.
    d. surgical consent is signed.

    Rationale: The answer is (d). Although the physician is responsible for obtaining the client's signature, it is most important for the nurse to ensure that it has been signed. Options (a), (b), and (c) are important but are not the most important answers.

1-24 WOUND ASSESSMENT

List the types of wounds:

1. _____

2. _____

List the types of wound drainage systems:

1. _____

2. _____

3. _____

4. _____

Match the **wound classifications and wound drainage terminology** with the appropriate description or characteristics:

1. Laceration
2. Contusion
3. Penetrating
4. Abrasion
5. Incision
6. Serosanguineous
7. Serous
8. Sanguineous
9. Purulent

____ Thin, clear, watery secretion
____ Containing pus
____ Open cut made with a knife/scalpel
____ Containing RBCs
____ Irregular wound tear; jagged edges
____ Entering into the tissues/body cavity
____ Closed wound; with pain, swelling, and discoloration
____ Red, watery secretion
____ A scraping away of the skin surface

CLINICAL SITUATION   Mr. J, 26 years old, received a stab wound to his abdomen and was taken to the emergency department. He underwent emergency surgery. He has an IV, nasogastric tube to continuous low wall suction, and one Jackson-Pratt on the right upper quadrant and another on the left lower quadrant of the abdomen. He has a closed abdominal wound and the dressing is clean and dry as he is taken to the surgical unit at 0800.

Pertinent Terminology	Definition
Primary Intention	_____
Secondary Intention	_____
Tertiary Intention	_____
Granulation Tissue	_____
Inflammatory Phase	_____
Proliferation Phase	_____
Maturation Phase	_____
Dehiscence	_____
Evisceration	_____

Use the clinical situation to **check off** (✓) all the factors that apply to Mr. J:

☐ High risk for infection

☐ Healing by secondary intention

☐ J-P will aid in the healing process

☐ Postop pain should initially increase

☐ J-P drainage should progressively decrease

☐ Slight redness around incision first day

At 1100, three hours after arriving in the surgical unit, the nurse took the vital signs and noted that Mr. J's surgical dressing has two abd pads and the dressing is currently saturated with sanguineous drainage. The nurse lightly palpated the abdomen.

Use the abd dressing image to implement appropriate nursing interventions.

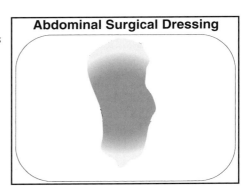

Abdominal Surgical Dressing

Select the nurse's documentation that demonstrates appropriate assessment:

___ Abdominal dressing with large amount of red drainage, abdomen tender, T 100.4°F

___ Abdominal dressing covered with pink reddish drainage, abdomen tender, no bowel sounds, P 88, BP 136/86

___ Abdominal dressing saturated with red drainage, abdomen tender, reinforced, P 88, BP 136/86

Collaborative Learning Activity: With a partner, use the statements below to (1) check (✓) whether the statement is correct or incorrect and (2) provide a rationale for your selection.

Statements	Correct/Incorrect	Rationale
1. Wound drainage devices need to be emptied once a shift.	☐ Correct ☐ Incorrect	
2. Wound drainage devices need to be compressed to function.	☐ Correct ☐ Incorrect	
3. Assessment of the wound should be done once a day.	☐ Correct ☐ Incorrect	
4. Wound description does not need to include wound measurement.	☐ Correct ☐ Incorrect	
5. Wound evisceration requires the application of sterile dry gauze.	☐ Correct ☐ Incorrect	

APPLYING CRITICAL THINKING SKILLS TO TEST QUESTIONS

INSTRUCTIONS: Circle the one best answer for each test question. Write your rationale for selecting the answer. To enhance your learning and test-taking skills, discuss your answer and rationale with a partner. The answer and the rationale can be found on the back of this page.

1. An elderly client is being discharged after abdominal surgery. The staples were removed on the third day after surgery and a gauze dressing was applied. The client tells the nurse that as he was standing up he heard a pop coming from his abdomen. Which nursing intervention is of priority?
   a. Fully assess the neurologic status of the client.
   b. Auscultate the bowel sounds.
   c. Assess the surgical site.
   d. Palpate the abdomen.

   Rationale for your selection: _____
   _____
   _____
   _____
   _____
   _____

2. On the second day after surgery, the nurse assesses a surgical wound and documents the following, "Surgical incision with stitches intact, erythema noted on surrounding skin around surgical incision, edges well approximated." On the basis of this documentation, the nurse most accurately assessed that the surgical wound:
   a. is healing without complications.
   b. is beginning to show signs of complications.
   c. needs to be assessed by the physician.
   d. will take longer to heal.

   Rationale for your selection: _____
   _____
   _____
   _____
   _____
   _____

3. In reviewing the patient's electronic health record, the nursing student collects the following data on the assigned patient who had abdominal surgery: abdominal dressing clean and dry, the J-P drainage output was 140 mL of red drainage on the day of surgery. On the first postop day, the abdominal dressing was changed by the physician and the total J-P drainage output was 100 mL of serosanguineous drainage. On the second post-op day, the total J-P output was 80 mL serosanguineous drainage. Based on these findings, which clinical judgment is most appropriate?
   a. The J-P drainage device will need to be emptied at the end of the shift.
   b. The J-P drainage device has not been compressed properly.
   c. Prepare the patient for removal of the drainage device.
   d. Decreased drainage is a part of the healing process.

   Rationale for your selection: _____
   _____
   _____
   _____
   _____

ANSWER KEY FOR
APPLYING CRITICAL THINKING SKILLS TO TEST QUESTIONS

HELPFUL HINTS: Read all test questions carefully. Identify key words in the question that will guide you in answering the question. In these test questions the **key words** to consider are **"priority," "most accurately,"** and **"most appropriate."** Compare your rationale with the one found for each question.

1. An elderly client is being discharged after abdominal surgery. The staples were removed on the third day after surgery and a gauze dressing was applied. The client tells the nurse that as he was standing up he heard a pop coming from his abdomen. Which nursing intervention is of priority?
   a. Fully assess the neurologic status of the client.
   b. Auscultate the bowel sounds.
   (c.) Assess the surgical site.
   d. Palpate the abdomen.

   Rationale: The answer is (c). Wound dehiscence is a possible complication and clients may not have any pain. With option (a) not enough data are present to suggest that a full neurologic assessment is warranted, and options (b) and (d) should be done after inspection.

2. On the second day after surgery, the nurse assesses a surgical wound and documents the following, "Surgical incision with stitches intact, erythema noted on surrounding skin around surgical incision, edges well approximated." On the basis of this documentation, the nurse most accurately assessed that the surgical wound:
   (a.) is healing without complications.
   b. is beginning to show signs of complications.
   c. needs to be assessed by the physician.
   d. will take longer to heal.

   Rationale: The answer is (a). Documentation describes the normal healing process of a second postoperative day surgical wound. Options (b), (c), and (d) are not appropriate at this time.

3. In reviewing the patient's electronic health record, the nursing student collects the following data on the assigned patient who had abdominal surgery: abdominal dressing clean and dry, the J-P drainage output was 140 mL of red drainage on the day of surgery. On the first postop day, the abdominal dressing was changed by the physician and the total J-P drainage output was 100 mL of serosanguineous drainage. On the second postop day, the total J-P output was 80 mL serosanguineous drainage. Based on these findings, which clinical judgment is most appropriate?
   a. The J-P drainage device will need to be emptied at the end of the shift.
   b. The J-P drainage device has not been compressed properly.
   c. Prepare the patient for removal of the drainage device.
   (d.) Decreased drainage is a part of the healing process.

   Rationale: The answer is (d). The amount of drainage decreases as the wound heals. Option (a) does not address the need to assess and empty the device as needed throughout the shift. Option (b) is not correct because the drainage has been recorded. Option (c) is not appropriate because the physician will determine the appropriate time for the removal of the J-P device.

1-25 WOUND DRESSINGS

List five basic wound dressings:

1. _____
2. _____
3. _____
4. _____
5. _____

Identify the purpose for using each type of dressing in wound management.

Alginate: _____
_____

Hydrogel: _____
_____

Hydrocolloid: _____
_____

Transparent film dressings: _____
_____
_____

Wet-dry gauze dressing: _____
_____
_____

CLINICAL SITUATION   Mr. Y, 78 years old, has been in the acute care setting for 2 months. He was admitted with a fractured left hip, anorexia, and weight loss. He has a stage IV pressure ulcer on the sacrum with undermining at 12 o'clock to 2 o'clock and eschar on the right heel. The physician orders: irrigate the sacral wound with normal saline solution, apply a hydrocolloid dressing to the sacrum, and change every 3–5 days.

Pertinent Terminology	Definition
Debridement	_____
	_____
Exudate	_____
	_____
Macerate	_____
	_____
Mechanical Debridement	_____
Wound Irrigation	_____
	_____
Wet-Dry	_____
	_____
	_____
Negative Pressure Wound Therapy (NPWT)	_____
	_____
	_____
Periwound Skin	_____
Tunneling	_____
	_____
Undermining	_____

The nurse is preparing to irrigate and apply the dressing on the sacral wound. Select all the statements that apply to wound irrigation and to the expected benefits of the hydrocolloid dressing.

Wound Irrigation	Sacral Hydrocolloid Dressing
☐ Clean the wound bed with iodine	☐ Protects periwound skin.
☐ Use a 35-mL syringe	☐ Can absorb large quantities of exudate.
☐ Irrigate with 0.9% normal saline solution	☐ Maintains a moist wound environment.
☐ Use a 3-mL syringe with a 22-gauge needle	☐ Removes necrotic tissue.
☐ Attach an 18-gauge angiocath to the irrigating syringe	☐ Requires another dry dressing to secure in place.

⚠️

The nurse writes the following data on the clinical worksheet:

Sacral wound
0900 Size 3.5 cm by 4.0 cm, irregular margins. Pressure ulcer 2.5 cm deep. Slough at margins. Tan-colored drainage moderate amount. Checked for undermining. Undermining at 12 o'clock to 2 o'clock. Hydrocolloid dressing applied. Irrigated with saline solution with a large syringe. Medicated with analgesic 30 minutes before procedure. Tolerated well.

Right heel wound
0900 Eschar on right heel. No changes from the previous notation 3 days ago.

Collaborative Learning Activity: With a partner, discuss the wound assessment observations made by the nurse. For the **sacral wound,** rewrite the assessment observations in the space provided.

For the **right heel wound,** identify why the documentation made by the nurse is *not* appropriate.

1-26 THE PATIENT WITH FLUID AND ELECTROLYTE IMBALANCE

List the **adult normal values** for the following electrolytes:

1. Sodium (Na^+) = _____

2. Potassium (K^+) = _____

3. Chloride (Cl^-) = _____

4. Calcium (Ca^{++}) = _____

5. Phosphate (PO_4^{-3}) = _____

6. Magnesium (Mg^{++}) = _____

Write in the appropriate medical terminology for the serum laboratory values below:

Mg^{++} 3.5 mg/dL = _____

K^+ 2.5 mEq/L   = _____

Cl^- 90 mEq/L   = _____

Na^+ 132 mEq/L   = _____

Ca^{++} 8.5 mg/dL = _____

PO_4^{-3} 5.1 mg/dL = _____

CLINICAL SITUATION   A 36-year-old client was admitted with gastroenteritis. He has been vomiting and having severe diarrhea for 2 days. He is very weak. The current laboratory results are Na^+ 128 mEq/L, K^+ 2.8 mEq/L, and Cl^- 90 mEq/L. The physician orders an IV of 0.9% sodium chloride with 20 mEq KCL at 100 mL/hr, NPO, and I & O.

Pertinent Terminology	Definition
Sodium (Na^+)	_____
Potassium (K^+)	_____
Chloride (Cl^-)	_____
Calcium (Ca^{++})	_____
Phosphate (PO_4^{-3})	_____
Magnesium (Mg^{++})	_____
Third Space	_____
Edema	_____
Pitting Edema	_____

From the clinical situation, identify the abnormal laboratory results. List the **major clinical signs or symptoms** that you would assess with each abnormal value:

_____   =   _____

_____

_____   =   _____

_____

_____   =   _____

_____

FOLLOW-UP CLINICAL SITUATION   The client's vomiting and diarrhea has begun to subside in the evening, and the MD has ordered a clear liquid diet. The client's **24-hour I & O** for the day is noted below:

24-Hour Intake/Output Record

IV	=	2400	Emesis	=	950
Oral	=	120	Diarrhea	=	900
			Urine	=	750
		2520 mL			2600 mL

On the basis of the clinical situation and intake and output record, **select** the most appropriate **NANDA-I nursing diagnoses** for the client:

____ Excess fluid volume   ____ Deficient fluid volume

____ Diarrhea   ____ Impaired skin integrity

____ Imbalanced nutrition: less than   ____ Risk for injury
body requirements

Collaborative Learning Activity: With a partner, read the following clinical situation and write a rationale for each of the nursing interventions listed.

Clinical Situation	Nursing Interventions	Rationale
Ms. M was admitted with heart failure. The nursing diagnosis of "Fluid volume excess r/t noncompliance to dietary Na^+ restriction" is listed in her NCP. Digoxin 0.25 mg qAM po, furosemide 40 mg qAM po, and potassium chloride tabs 10 mEq po tid are her medications.	Weigh daily	
	Monitor I & O	
	Take apical pulse	
	Assess skin	
	Assess lungs	
	Assess for peripheral edema	
	✓ Neck veins	

1-27 ELIMINATION – URINARY

List the **factors** that affect bladder elimination:

1. _____
2. _____
3. _____
4. _____
5. _____
6. _____
7. _____
8. _____
9. _____

Use the diagrams to **select** the appropriate size of the indwelling catheter for the female and male patient. **Draw a line** on the catheter at the anticipated length of insertion.

Female

14 fr

18 fr

Male

20 fr

16 fr

CLINICAL SITUATION   Mrs. S, a 42-year-old woman, had abdominal surgery 2 days ago. She has an IV infusing into her left forearm, an indwelling urinary catheter (Foley), and she has a temperature of 100.4°F this evening. She states her pain level is about 2 out of 10. The physician orders the indwelling catheter to be removed in the AM.

Pertinent Terminology	Definition
UA	_____
Nocturia	_____
Hematuria	_____
Dysuria	_____
Oliguria	_____
Anuria	_____
Urinary Incontinence	_____
Residual Urine	_____
Midstream UA	_____
Void	_____
Indwelling Catheter	_____
Condom Catheter	_____

Using the information in the clinical situation, the nurse gathers more information and documents on Mrs. S's chart. **Select the statement** below that describes a thorough observation of the urinary system:

1. Indwelling catheter patent to gravity, taking fluids liberally.

2. Indwelling catheter to gravity, draining cloudy, pale yellow urine.

3. Indwelling catheter patent to gravity, output 75 mL.

4. Indwelling catheter patent, draining freely; abdomen without distention.

⚠ The next morning, the nurse prepares to remove the indwelling catheter. Identify the equipment the nurse needs to gather to properly remove the catheter.

_____

The indwelling catheter is removed at 0800. The nurse knows that Mrs. S should void within _____ hours after removal of the catheter.

⚙ **Collaborative Learning Activity:** With a partner, **select the NANDA-I nursing diagnosis** most appropriate to the clinical situations below that describe the complications Mrs. S had after removal of the indwelling catheter.

NANDA-I nursing diagnoses: (1) Stress urinary incontinence   (2) Urinary retention
(3) Impaired urinary elimination   (4) Risk for infection

Clinical Situation	Nursing Diagnosis
Mrs. S is unable to void 6 hours after removal of the indwelling catheter. She has abdominal discomfort, a sensation of fullness, and frequent dribbling.	
Mrs. S is catheterized for residual urine and 700 mL of urine are drained from the bladder. An indwelling catheter is left in place again.	
The following day the catheter is removed. Mrs. S is able to void without any further problems that day. The next day she complains of frequency and dysuria when she voids.	
Mrs. S is prescribed an antibiotic. She notices that the dysuria and hematuria are no longer present. However, she tells you that she has a history of leaking urine when she coughs or sneezes.	

APPLYING CRITICAL THINKING SKILLS TO TEST QUESTIONS

INSTRUCTIONS: Circle the one best answer for each test question. Write your rationale for selecting the answer. To enhance your learning and test-taking skills, discuss your answer and rationale with a partner. The answer and the rationale can be found on the back of this page.

1. The physician writes the following order on admission for an adult female patient, "Insert Foley catheter stat." It is most appropriate for the nurse to initially insert a:
   a. 14 F catheter.
   b. 16 F catheter.
   c. 20 F catheter.
   d. 22 F catheter.

   Rationale for your selection: _____
   _____
   _____
   _____
   _____
   _____

2. The nurse is caring for a client who has a urinary catheter. To accurately assess the urine color, it is most important for the nurse to:
   a. look at the color and amount of urine in the drainage bag.
   b. draw 1 to 2 mL of urine from the catheter port.
   c. look at the color of the urine in the drainage tube.
   d. review the color of the urine recorded by the previous shift.

   Rationale for your selection: _____
   _____
   _____
   _____
   _____
   _____

3. The physician writes the following order: "I & O cath for residual this AM." Which statement, given to a nursing assistant by the nurse, is most helpful for implementing this order?
   a. "Let me know when the client wants to void."
   b. "Let me know as soon as the client voids."
   c. "Push fluids this morning."
   d. "Record how much the client voids this morning."

   Rationale for your selection: _____
   _____
   _____
   _____
   _____
   _____

ANSWER KEY FOR
APPLYING CRITICAL THINKING SKILLS TO TEST QUESTIONS

HELPFUL HINTS: Read all test questions carefully. Identify key words in the question that will guide you in answering the question. In these test questions the **key words** to consider are **"most appropriate," "accurately assess," "most important,"** and **"most helpful."** Compare your rationale with the one in the test question.

1. The physician writes the following order on admission for an adult female patient, "Insert Foley catheter stat." It is most appropriate for the nurse to initially insert a:
   a. 14 F catheter.
   b. 16 F catheter.
   c. 20 F catheter.
   d. 22 F catheter.

   Rationale: The answer is (a). The nurse will insert the smallest catheter to avoid trauma and unnecessary dilation of the urethra. Option (b) can be used if a 14 F catheter is not available. Options (c) and (d) are too large in diameter for a routine catheterization.

2. The nurse is caring for a client who has a urinary catheter. To accurately assess the urine color, it is most important for the nurse to:
   a. look at the color and amount of urine in the drainage bag.
   b. draw 1 to 2 mL of urine from the catheter port.
   c. look at the color of the urine in the drainage tube.
   d. review the color of the urine recorded by the previous shift.

   Rationale: The answer is (c). The color of the urine is best noted in the drainage tube because the tube contains the most recent urine coming from the bladder. Option (b) is used to obtain a urine specimen, option (a) is not the best because urine collecting in the bag may look darker, and option (d) does not provide the most current assessment of the urine.

3. The physician writes the following order: "I & O cath for residual this AM." Which statement, given to a nursing assistant by the nurse, is most helpful for implementing this order?
   a. "Let me know when the client wants to void."
   b. "Let me know as soon as the client voids."
   c. "Push fluids this morning."
   d. "Record how much the client voids this morning."

   Rationale: The answer is (b). Catheterizing for residual requires that the procedure be implemented as soon as the client voids. This will provide information as to the amount of urine left in the bladder after the client has voided. Options (a), (c), and (d) do not address the directions needed for implementing the order.

1-28 ELIMINATION – BOWEL

List the **factors** that affect bowel elimination:

1. _____
2. _____
3. _____
4. _____
5. _____
6. _____
7. _____

Use the diagram to identify the location and placement of the stethoscope when listening for bowel sounds. Draw a **circle** at each location.

CLINICAL SITUATION The physician notes the following from the history and physical form after examining a 55-year-old client, Mr. M: Complains of cramping abdominal pain, borborygmi, 5–6 dark brown semi-liquid BMs per day for several days. Last bowel movement this AM. Indicates no changes in diet intake. Denies melena, constipation, nausea, or vomiting. The MD orders an upper endoscopy, barium enema, and stool for occult blood.

Pertinent Terminology	Definition
Bowel Sounds	
Flatus	
Constipation	
Diarrhea	
Occult Blood	
Melena	
Enema	
Fecal Impaction	
Borborygmi	
Upper Endoscopy	
Barium Enema	

Using the information identified in the history and physical, identify the questions that the nurse could ask
Mr. M to **assess** the bowel pattern changes that he is currently experiencing:

1. Complains of cramping abdominal pain, borborygmi

   Question: _____

2. 5–6 dark brown semiliquid BMs per day for several days

   Question: _____

3. Indicates no changes in diet intake

   Question: _____

4. Denies melena, constipation, nausea, or vomiting

   Question: _____

5. Last bowel movement this AM

   Question: _____

Write two questions that would be useful in further assessing Mr. M's bowel function:

1. _____

2. _____

Discuss how these questions contribute to the assessment.

Collaborative Learning Activity: With a partner, select the NANDA-I nursing diagnosis that best
applies to each of the clinical situations below:

NANDA-I nursing diagnoses: (1) Perceived constipation   (2) Diarrhea
                             (3) Constipation   (4) Bowel incontinence

Clinical Situation	Nursing Diagnosis
The client takes a mild laxative every night since his retirement 1 year ago. He believes that his change in activity will cause him bowel problems.	
The client was in a car accident 1 month ago in which she sustained a neuromuscular back injury. While hospitalized she was having involuntary frequent loose BMs.	
The nursing diagnosis for Mr. M in the clinical situation is:	

1-29 GENERAL NUTRITION

A therapeutic diet is defined as:

_____

_____

List the most common methods for providing enteral nutrition:

1. _____
2. _____
3. _____

Circle the letter of the therapeutic diet where the foods/fluids may be served.

Clear Liquid (C)   Full Liquid (F)   Soft (S)

Custard	C	F	S
Cook vegetables	C	F	S
Juices with pulp	C	F	S
Strained cream soups	C	F	S
Juices without pulp	C	F	S
Cooked cereals	C	F	S
Ice cream	C	F	S
Eggs	C	F	S
Broth	C	F	S
Tea/Coffee without milk	C	F	S
Honey	C	F	S
Gelatin	C	F	S
Tuna fish	C	F	S

CLINICAL SITUATION   A 68-year-old male client had a cerebral vascular accident 2 weeks ago. He has right-sided hemiplegia. The patient care plan indicates that the client is on a soft pureed diet with thickened liquids and is on intake and output.

Pertinent Terminology	Definition
Regular Diet	_____
Soft Diet	_____
Full Liquid	_____
Clear Liquid	_____
Pureed	_____
Enteral Nutrition	_____
Gastric Gavage	_____
Nasogastric Tube	_____
PEG	_____
Jejunostomy Tube	_____

Use the information from the clinical situation to **mark an "X"** on the most appropriate feeding guidelines for the client who has right-sided hemiplegia:

Feeding Guidelines

☐ Give water frequently with the food
☐ Check right cheek for "pocketing"
☐ Place in semi-Fowler's position
☐ Teach and allow family to feed Mr. G

☐ Place in high Fowler's position
☐ Give thickened juices
☐ Provide oral care
☐ Lie flat after feeding

⚙ Collaborative Learning Activity: With a partner, use the clinical situations related to the client. For each situation, **prioritize the NANDA-I nursing diagnosis. #1** = Priority, **#2** = Important, and **#3** = Need to monitor.

Clinical Situation	NANDA-I Nursing Diagnosis
The client's intake for last 24 hrs = 1250 mL and his output = 725 mL. He is fatigued and needs to be reminded to drink and eat. His skin is dry and flaky. Skin turgor—tenting. Oral mucous membranes dry, swallows with difficulty, several teeth missing. Urine color is dark yellow.	— Deficient fluid volume related to fatigue and forgetting to eat and drink. — Impaired oral mucous membranes as evidenced by insufficient intake of fluids. — Risk for impaired skin integrity as evidenced by dry, thin, fragile skin.
The client has frequent episodes of coughing forcefully while being fed during meals. The feedings were stopped and the MD ordered for him to be NPO. The client has lost 3 lbs in 1 week. He has an IV of D5W infusing at 75 mL/hr. It is difficult to get him out of bed because he is weak and does not assist with the transfer.	— Imbalanced nutrition: less than body requirements related to inability to ingest food as evidenced by having difficulty swallowing. — Risk for aspiration as evidenced by difficulty swallowing food. — Risk for impaired skin integrity as evidenced by prolonged bed rest and weakness.
The nurse is planning the care of a client who suffered a heart attack 6 months ago and is admitted for diagnostic tests. The client is hypertensive and has not been following the recommended low cholesterol diet because "it is too difficult." The client does not like the food served in the hospital and requests that his family bring in food from home.	— Ineffective health management related to not following prescribed diet as evidenced by verbalizing diet is difficult to maintain. — Deficient knowledge related to following prescribed diet as evidenced by not eating recommended diet. — Risk for impaired cardiovascular function as evidenced by history of cardiovascular disease.

1-30 GASTROINTESTINAL TRACT

List the structures in the gastrointestinal tract involved with the digestion and absorption of food:

1. _____

2. _____

3. _____

4. _____

Use the diagram to **identify the quadrants** **(RLQ,RUQ,LLQ,LUQ)** and the **anatomic** **regions of the abdomen** (Right and Left Lumbar, Right and Left Inguinal, Umbilical, Epigastric, Suprapubic, and Right and Left Hypochondriac)

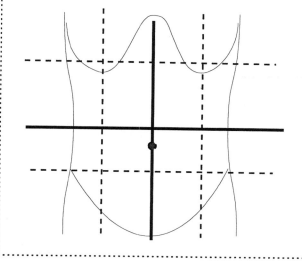

Modified from Black JM, Hawks JH, Keene AM: *Medical-surgical nursing: clinical management for positive outcomes,* ed 8, St. Louis, 2009, WB Saunders.

CLINICAL SITUATION   Mrs. T is a 55-year-old woman who was admitted to the hospital with complaints of diarrhea for the past 10 days. She states that she has abdominal cramping and at times passes bloody stools. She is scheduled for a colonoscopy at 10:00 AM today.

Pertinent Terminology	Definition
Duodenum	_____
Jejunum	_____
Ileum	_____
Cecum	_____
Colon	_____
Rectum	_____
Polyp	_____

Use the clinical situation to **check off (✓) all the nursing interventions and physician's orders** that you would associate with the preparation of Mrs. T for the colonoscopy procedure.

☐ NPO for procedure   ☐ Consent is necessary

☐ An osmotic bowel preparation will be given for stool evacuation   ☐ May have a clear liquid breakfast

☐ Monitor for abdominal pain and bleeding after the procedure   ☐ Requires general anesthesia

Match the gastrointestinal diagnostic test with the appropriate definition:

Diagnostic Test		Definition
1. Colonscopy	__	Visualization of the rectum and sigmoid
2. Endoscopy	__	Visualization from anus to cecum
3. Sigmoidoscopy	__	Visualization of esophagus, stomach, and small bowel
4. Barium swallow	__	Visualization of interior organs and structures using a fiberoptic instrument

⚙ Collaborative Learning Activity: With a partner, use the diagram to:

1. Identify the segments of the large intestine.
2. Follow the path of the colonoscopy procedure.
3. Identify the consistency of the stool as it moves through the intestinal tract (mushy, semiliquid, and solid).

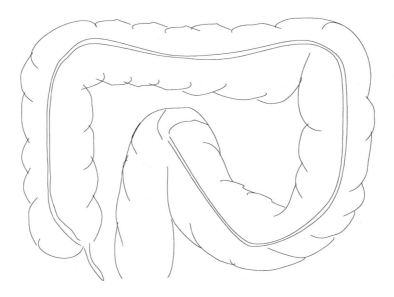

APPLYING CRITICAL THINKING SKILLS TO TEST QUESTIONS

INSTRUCTIONS: Circle the one best answer for each test question. Write your rationale for selecting the answer. To enhance your learning and test-taking skills, discuss your answer and rationale with a partner. The answer and the rationale can be found on the back of this page.

1. The client is scheduled for an upper endoscopy. Which statement is correct in providing the client with information about this endoscopic procedure?
   a. "A tube will be passed from your nose into your stomach."
   b. "The tube is small, very flexible, and has a light at the end."
   c. "The tube has a light that will allow the doctor to see your intestines."
   d. "A tube will be passed from your mouth and into your stomach."

   Rationale for your selection: _____
   _____
   _____
   _____
   _____
   _____

2. The day after having a barium enema as an outpatient, the client calls the clinic nurse to express concern because the stools are white in color. Which statement made by the nurse is most helpful?
   a. "Don't worry; this is normal after a barium enema."
   b. "This is expected; be sure to drink plenty of fluids."
   c. "The stool color should return after 1 to 2 days."
   d. "This is expected; call back if your stools are still white after 5 days."

   Rationale for your selection: _____
   _____
   _____
   _____
   _____
   _____

3. The nurse is taking care of a 76-year-old client who is having an upper gastrointestinal series this morning. After the completion of the procedure, the nurse should initially:
   a. see whether a laxative is ordered for the client.
   b. assess the bowel sounds.
   c. take the vital signs.
   d. observe for intestinal obstruction.

   Rationale for your selection: _____
   _____
   _____
   _____
   _____
   _____

ANSWER KEY FOR
APPLYING CRITICAL THINKING SKILLS TO TEST QUESTIONS

HELPFUL HINTS: Read all test questions carefully. Identify key words in the question that will guide you in answering the question. In these test questions the **key words** to consider are **"correct," "most helpful,"** and **"initially."** Compare your rationale with the one in the test question.

1. The client is scheduled for an upper endoscopy. Which statement is correct in providing the client with information about this endoscopic procedure?
   a. "A tube will be passed from your nose into your stomach."
   b. "The tube is small, very flexible, and has a light at the end."
   c. "The tube has a light that will allow the doctor to see your intestines."
   d. "A tube will be passed from your mouth and into your stomach."

   Rationale: The answer is (d). This is a beginning statement that informs the client as to how the procedure will be carried out. Options (a), (b), and (c) do not provide accurate information about the procedure.

2. The day after having a barium enema as an outpatient, the client calls the clinic nurse to express concern because the stools are white in color. Which statement made by the nurse is most helpful?
   a. "Don't worry; this is normal after a barium enema."
   b. "This is expected; be sure to drink plenty of fluids."
   c. "The stool color should return after 1 to 2 days."
   d. "This is expected; call back if your stools are still white after 5 days."

   Rationale: The answer is (b). It is important to reassure the client and to provide instructions that help minimize complications. Barium impaction is a concern after a barium enema. Options (a), (c), and (d) do not provide enough information.

3. The nurse is taking care of a 76-year-old client who is having an upper gastrointestinal series this morning. After the completion of the procedure, the nurse should initially:
   a. see whether a laxative is ordered for the client.
   b. assess the bowel sounds.
   c. take the vital signs.
   d. observe for intestinal obstruction.

   Rationale: The answer is (a). To prevent the complication of fecal impaction after an upper gastrointestinal series (barium swallow), a laxative is usually given after the procedure. Options (b) and (c) are good interventions, but the situation does not address the need for these interventions; option (d) does not focus on the initial intervention.

1-31 DIABETES MELLITUS

List the classic symptoms of diabetes mellitus:

1. _____
2. _____
3. _____
4. _____

List other **signs** and **symptoms** associated with **hyperglycemia:**

1. _____
2. _____
3. _____
4. _____
5. _____
6. _____
7. _____

Fill in the **circles** that identify the **signs and symptoms** associated with **hypoglycemia.**

O Polyuria   O Shakiness

O Tremor

O Behavior changes   O Glucosuria

O Polydipsia

O Sweating   O Confusion

O Dizziness   O Headache

O Hunger

O Slurred speech

O Paresthesia   O Tachycardia

CLINICAL SITUATION   A 20-year-old woman makes an appointment with her physician for complaints of feeling fatigued and lethargic for several days. She states that she has noticed that she has lost 15 lbs. She tells the physician that she does not understand why she has lost so much weight because she has been eating a lot. She indicates that she smokes e-cigarettes instead of regular cigarettes. The physician asks whether she voids more than usual. The client says that she does but thinks it is because of all the water that she is drinking all day.

Pertinent Terminology	Definition
Diabetes Mellitus (DM)	_____ _____
Type 1 Diabetes	_____ _____
Type 2 Diabetes	_____ _____
Insulin Resistance Insulin	_____ _____
Counterregulatory	_____ _____
Oral Hypoglycemic Agents	_____ _____ _____
Fasting Plasma Glucose (FPG) Casual Blood Glucose	_____ _____ _____
Glycosylate Hemoglobin A1C	_____ _____

The client's physician orders a fasting plasma glucose (FPG) test. Another FPG and a 2-hr oral glucose tolerance test (OGTT) and A1C are also ordered. The following results are noted in the client's clinic chart. **Write** the normal laboratory value for the test in the column provided.

Test	Results	Normal Laboratory Values
FPG	130 mg/dL	
FPG	160 mg/dL	
OGTT 2-hr postload glucose	225 mg/dL	
A1C	7.2%	

The client is informed that she has type 1 diabetes mellitus. **Fill in** the circles that correlate with the diagnosis and treatment of type 1 diabetes mellitus.

- ○ Oral hypoglycemics will be ordered
- ○ Exercise is part of the treatment plan
- ○ Will need to monitor for signs and symptoms of hypoglycemia
- ○ Insulin will be required every day

- ○ Will require blood glucose testing
- ○ Beta cells are producing insulin
- ○ Will need to monitor for signs and symptoms of hyperglycemia
- ○ Will not need insulin if follows diet

Collaborative Learning Activity: With a partner, match each question in the follow-up clinical situation with the appropriate response(s) in the Key Points Box. Next to each question, write the letter(s) of the responses you have selected.

Key Points Box

A. "Usually 30 min to 1 hr before breakfast."	E. "Destroyed by the gastric enzymes."
B. "Insulin needs may change over time."	F. "No."
C. "Check blood sugar level."	G. "Drink apple or grape juice."
D. "Always carry oral glucose tablets."	H. "Know the signs and symptoms of hypoglycemia."

FOLLOW-UP CLINICAL SITUATION The client is prescribed on isophane NPH insulin 15 units qAM, and isophane NPH insulin 5 units qPM. She is taught how to do self-monitoring blood glucose checks (SMBG) qid.

Client's Questions	Responses
1. "When is the best time to administer the AM insulin?"	
2. "If I forget the PM dose of insulin, can I double the dose in the morning?"	
3. "What should I do if I begin to get shaky and dizzy?"	
4. "How do I prepare for a hypoglycemic reaction?"	

APPLYING CRITICAL THINKING SKILLS TO TEST QUESTIONS

INSTRUCTIONS: Circle the one best answer for each test question. Write your rationale for selecting the answer. To enhance your learning and test-taking skills, discuss your answer and rationale with a partner. The answer and the rationale can be found on the back of this page.

1. A client is diagnosed with diabetes mellitus type 1. In teaching the client about diabetes mellitus type 1, it is most important for the client to:
   a. know how to use oral hypoglycemic agents.
   b. understand that insulin injections will be required daily.
   c. randomly check fingerstick blood glucose throughout the day.
   d. decrease physical activity.

   Rationale for your selection: _____
   _____
   _____
   _____
   _____
   _____

2. The nurse learns during the handoff morning report that the 0700 fasting blood glucose of a client was 72 mg/dL. Which of the following morning assessment findings is of priority?
   a. Abdominal wound dressing with moderate dried red drainage.
   b. Complaining of thirst and dried mouth.
   c. Output of 250 mL during the night shift.
   d. Diaphoresis noted while taking vital signs.

   Rationale for your selection: _____
   _____
   _____
   _____
   _____
   _____

3. The nurse is assigned to a client who has just been diagnosed with diabetes mellitus type 1. Which of the following assessment findings is most consistent with this diagnosis?
   a. FPG 110 mg/dL, hypertension, decreased urinary output.
   b. Casual blood glucose of 140 mg/dL, obese, limited physical activity.
   c. Weight loss, episodes of shakiness and diaphoresis.
   d. Frequent urination, hunger, and excessive fluid intake.

   Rationale for your selection: _____
   _____
   _____
   _____
   _____
   _____

ANSWER KEY FOR
APPLYING CRITICAL THINKING SKILLS TO TEST QUESTIONS

HELPFUL HINTS: Read all test questions carefully. Identify key words in the question that will guide you in answering the question. In these test questions the **key words** to consider are **"most important," "priority,"** and **"most consistent."** Compare your rationale with the one in the test question.

1. A client is diagnosed with diabetes mellitus type 1. In teaching the client about diabetes mellitus type 1, it is most important for the client to:
   a. know how to use oral hypoglycemic agents.
   b. understand that insulin injections will be required daily.
   c. randomly check fingerstick blood glucose throughout the day.
   d. decrease physical activity.

   Rationale: The answer is (b). With diabetes mellitus type 1, the beta cells have stopped functioning and the use of exogenous insulin administration is required. Option (a) is not appropriate for type 1 diabetes mellitus because hypoglycemic oral agents are used for type 2 DM. Option (c) is incorrect because blood glucose is monitored at specific times for control; option (d) is incorrect because exercise is recommended.

2. The nurse learns during the handoff morning report that the 0700 fasting blood glucose of a client was 72 mg/dL. Which of the following morning assessment findings is of priority?
   a. Abdominal wound dressing with moderate dried red drainage.
   b. Complaining of thirst and dried mouth.
   c. Output of 250 mL during the night shift.
   d. Diaphoresis noted while taking vital signs.

   Rationale: The answer is (d). Diaphoresis is a sign associated with hypoglycemia and should be assessed further. Also, the morning blood glucose was toward the lower limit of normal. Options (a) and (c) are within normal limits, and option (b) is important but not a priority.

3. The nurse is assigned to a client who has just been diagnosed with diabetes mellitus type 1. Which of the following assessment findings is most consistent with this diagnosis?
   a. FPG 110 mg/dL, hypertension, decreased urinary output.
   b. Casual blood glucose of 140 mg/dL, obese, limited physical activity.
   c. Weight loss, episodes of shakiness, and diaphoresis.
   d. Frequent urination, hunger, and excessive fluid intake.

   Rationale: The answer is (d). The classic signs and symptoms associated with diabetes mellitus type 1 are polyuria, polydipsia, and polyphagia. Options (a), (b), and (c) are not the most consistent with the diagnosis.

1-32 COMPLICATIONS OF DIABETES MELLITUS

List the **causes** that precipitate **hypoglycemic reactions:**

1. _____

2. _____

3. _____

4. _____

5. _____

List the **causes** that precipitate the development of **diabetic ketoacidosis:**

1. _____

2. _____

3. _____

For each line identify a specific **long-term complication,** eg, stroke, associated with diabetes mellitus.

Diabetes Mellitus

CLINICAL SITUATION   Mr. E, 56 years old, has been a diabetic for 25 years. He is admitted to the hospital after having a cerebral vascular accident (CVA). His wife says that her husband monitors his blood glucose daily and administers his own insulin. However, she tells the nurse that he does not always stick to his diet. She wonders whether this may have contributed to the CVA. Mr. E has an order for isophane NPH insulin 36 units qAM and isophane NPH insulin 12 units qPM with fingerstick blood glucose checks ac and hour of sleep. He is started on a correction insulin scale (sliding scale insulin).

Pertinent Terminology	Definition
Lipoatrophy	_____
Lipohypertrophy	_____
Impaired Fasting Glucose	_____
Dawn Phenomenon	_____
Diabetic Ketoacidosis (DKA)	_____
Hyperglycemic Hyperosmolar Nonketotic Syndrome (HHNS)	_____
Correction Insulin Scale (Sliding Scale Insulin)	_____

Use the **clinical situation, the follow-up information, and the nursing interventions below** to plan out Mr. E's morning care in the order of **priority.** Place a number, beginning with 1, in each box to indicate the sequence of the nursing care that should be delivered by the nurse.

Follow-up information: The AM blood glucose fingerstick and insulin are to be done by the morning shift. Mr. E is started on a diet containing semithick liquids.

	Nursing Interventions	Rationale
	Perform a body systems assessment	
	Perform a fingerstick	
	Take the AM vital signs	
	Administer morning insulin	
	Perform morning care	
	Provide information regarding the complications of diabetes	
	Assist with breakfast	

Place a check (✓) next to the statements that are correct regarding the use of a correction insulin scale (sliding scale).

☐ Regular or rapid-acting insulin is used   ☐ Used for patients with diabetes mellitus type 1

☐ Dosage based on ac blood glucose levels   ☐ Used for patients with diabetes mellitus type 2

☐ May be mixed with all other insulins   ☐ Used during periods of illness

Collaborative Learning Activity: The following nursing diagnosis is found on Mr. E's plan of care. With a partner, write the three most important nursing interventions for the risk for nursing diagnosis.

Nursing Diagnosis	Nursing Interventions
Risk for unstable blood glucose level as evidenced by the compromised (CVA) health status	1.
	2.
	3.

APPLYING CRITICAL THINKING SKILLS TO TEST QUESTIONS

INSTRUCTIONS: Circle the one best answer for each test question. Write your rationale for selecting the answer. To enhance your learning and test-taking skills, discuss your answer and rationale with a partner. The answer and the rationale can be found on the back of this page.

1. The nurse notes that the assigned client has an AV fistula on the right arm and is scheduled for hemodialysis this morning. In delegating the care of the client, it is most important for the nurse to:
   a. inform the nursing assistant to give the bath after the hemodialysis.
   b. direct that all morning care be done before hemodialysis.
   c. instruct that the blood pressure be taken on the left arm.
   d. ask that the client be weighed first.

   Rationale for your selection: _____
   _____
   _____
   _____
   _____
   _____

2. The nurse is preparing to administer 0.36 mL of a drug. Select the syringe that most accurately measures this dose.
   a. 5-mL syringe
   b. 3-mL syringe
   c. 2.5-mL syringe
   d. 1-mL syringe

   Rationale for your selection: _____
   _____
   _____
   _____
   _____
   _____

3. The nurse is taking care of a client who has diabetes mellitus type 1. The client tells the nurse that he is beginning to feel shaky and is experiencing symptoms of hypoglycemia. Which action by the nurse is of priority?
   a. Have the client drink a glass of apple juice.
   b. Monitor for signs of hypoglycemia.
   c. Take the pulse, respiration, and blood pressure.
   d. Have the laboratory perform a blood glucose test stat.

   Rationale for your selection: _____
   _____
   _____
   _____
   _____
   _____

ANSWER KEY FOR
APPLYING CRITICAL THINKING SKILLS TO TEST QUESTIONS

HELPFUL HINTS: Read all test questions carefully. Identify key words in the question that will guide you in answering the question. In these test questions the **key words** to consider are **"most important"** and **"priority."** Compare your rationale with the one in the test question.

1. The nurse notes that the assigned client has an AV fistula on the right arm and is scheduled for hemodialysis this morning. In delegating the care of the client, it is most important for the nurse to:
   a. inform the nursing assistant to give the bath after the hemodialysis.
   b. direct that all morning care be done before hemodialysis.
   c. instruct that the blood pressure be taken on the left arm.
   d. ask that the client be weighed first.

   Rationale: The answer is (c). It is most important to ensure the patency of the AV fistula and prevent vascular complications that can occur with applied pressure from the BP cuff. Options (a) and (b) can be done anytime, and although option (d) is important, it is not the most important on the basis of this situation.

2. The nurse is preparing to administer 0.36 mL of a drug. Select the syringe that most accurately measures this dose.
   a. 5-mL syringe
   b. 3-mL syringe
   c. 2.5-mL syringe
   d. 1-mL syringe

   Rationale: The answer is (d). The 1 mL syringe is calibrated to measure to the hundredths place accurately. Options (a), (b), and (c) are calibrated to measure to the tenths place and therefore will not accurately measure a dose calculated to the hundredths place.

3. The nurse is taking care of a client who has diabetes mellitus type 1. The client tells the nurse that he is beginning to feel shaky and is experiencing symptoms of hypoglycemia. Which action by the nurse is of priority?
   a. Have the client drink a glass of apple juice.
   b. Monitor for signs of hypoglycemia.
   c. Take the pulse, respiration, and blood pressure.
   d. Have the laboratory perform a blood glucose test stat.

   Rationale: The answer is (a). The hypoglycemic effects can occur rapidly. It is always better to treat hypoglycemia in the early stages, before there are signs of central nervous system involvement. Options (b), (c), and (d) do not focus on the immediate treatment.

1-33 INSULIN THERAPY

List the **onset**, **peak**, and **duration** of the following insulins:

Rapid-acting:
Onset _____
Peak _____
Duration _____

Short-acting:
Onset _____
Peak _____
Duration _____

Intermediate-acting:
Onset _____
Peak _____
Duration _____

Long-acting:
Onset _____
Peak _____
Duration _____

In the boxes in the left column write **(R)** if the insulin is rapid acting, **(S)** if the insulin is short acting, **(I)** if the insulin is intermediate acting, and **(L)** if the insulin is long acting.

	Insulin glargine	
	50% insulin lispro protamine suspension and 50% insulin lispro injection	
	Regular human insulin	
	Isophane insulin NPH	
	Human lispro	
	Insulin aspart	
	Insulin glulisine	
	Insulin detemir	

In the boxes on the right side, place an **"X"** to identify the insulin that may be given **IV.**

CLINICAL SITUATION Marty, 22 years old, has been on isophane NPH insulin since her diagnosis of type 1 diabetes mellitus 2 years ago. Marty administers 12 units isophane NPH insulin with 5 units regular human insulin qAM and 4 units isophane NPH insulin qPM. She monitors her blood glucose qid AC and before bedtime and routinely administers the AM insulin dose at 0700 and the PM dose at 1700. Marty maintains a daily chart of her blood glucose results. The latest A1C result is 7%.

Pertinent Terminology	Definition
Glucagon	_____
Glycogenolysis Gluconeogenesis	_____
Basal Insulin	_____
Bolus Insulin	_____
Hypoglycemia	_____
Insulin Analogs	_____

From the clinical situation, plot out Marty's morning dose of isophane NPH insulin and regular human insulin on the **Insulin Progression Graph**. Begin with the **onset (O)**, followed by identifying the **peak of action (P)** of the insulin, and the **duration (D)**.

Insulin Progression Graph
Onset → Peak → Duration

Length of time insulin remains in the body

| P | 0700 | 0800 | 0900 | 1000 | 1100 | 1200 | 1300 | 1400 | 1500 | 1600 | 1700 | 1800 | 1900 | 2000 | 2100 | 2200 | 2300 | 2400 | 0100 | 0200 | 0300 | 0400 | 0500 | 0600 |

D

O

↑ AM   Humulin N and Humalin R insulin administered

Marty eats a full breakfast at 0800 but is unable to eat lunch. Use the **Insulin Progression Graph** to indicate the time Marty would most likely experience a **hypoglycemic episode.** _____

Select (✓) the most appropriate **snack** for Marty to eat if she experiences a hypoglycemic reaction at 1600 and has a fingerstick blood glucose of 64 mg/dL.

_____ 6 saltine crackers

_____ 4 oz apple juice

_____ 8 oz diet soda

Collaborative Learning Activity: With a partner, **underline** the **correct word** in each statement as it relates to the sentence and provide a rationale for your selection.

1. For the patient with diabetes mellitus type 1, moderate exercise may have **hyperglycemic** or **hypoglycemic** effects.

   Rationale: _____

   _____

2. A patient with diabetes mellitus type 1 performs a fingerstick before exercising, and the blood glucose result is 92 mg/dL. The patient should eat a snack **before** or **immediately after** exercising.

   Rationale: _____

   _____

3. Excess alcohol consumption puts the patient with diabetes mellitus type 1 at risk for **hypoglycemia** or **hyperglycemia.**

   Rationale: _____

   _____

APPLYING CRITICAL THINKING SKILLS TO TEST QUESTIONS

INSTRUCTIONS: Circle the one best answer for each test question. Write your rationale for selecting the answer. To enhance your learning and test-taking skills, discuss your answer and rationale with a partner. The answer and the rationale can be found on the back of this page.

1. The nurse learns during the handoff report that the assigned client has a fingerstick blood glucose result of 100 mg/dL at 0700. The client receives isophane NPH insulin 15 units subcut qAM. On the basis of the morning handoff report, it is most appropriate for the nurse to:
   a. hold the AM dose of insulin.
   b. administer the AM dose of insulin.
   c. call the physician to report the blood glucose results.
   d. repeat the fingerstick blood glucose test at 0800.

   Rationale for your selection: _____
   _____
   _____
   _____
   _____
   _____

2. The physician orders isophane NPH insulin 23 units subcut qAM. The nurse carries out this order correctly when the insulin:
   a. dose is given after breakfast.
   b. dose is based on the fingerstick blood glucose results.
   c. is given according to the hospital's qAM schedule.
   d. is administered before breakfast.

   Rationale for your selection: _____
   _____
   _____
   _____
   _____
   _____

3. A client with diabetes mellitus type 1 has a correction insulin scale (sliding scale) with regular human insulin listed in the electronic medication record. Based on this finding, it is most important for the nurse to:
   a. administer the regular human insulin on the basis of the fasting blood glucose level.
   b. monitor the client's urine for ketones before meals.
   c. obtain fingerstick blood glucose test before meals.
   d. check the fingerstick blood glucose qid.

   Rationale for your selection: _____
   _____
   _____
   _____
   _____
   _____

ANSWER KEY FOR
APPLYING CRITICAL THINKING SKILLS TO TEST QUESTIONS

HELPFUL HINTS: Read all test questions carefully. Identify key words in the question that will guide you in answering the question. In these test questions the **key words** to consider are **"most appropriate," "correctly,"** and **"most important."** Compare your rationale with the one in the test question.

1. The nurse learns during the handoff report that the assigned client has a fingerstick blood glucose result of 100 mg/dL at 0700. The client receives isophane NPH insulin 15 units subcut qAM. On the basis of the morning handoff report, it is most appropriate for the nurse to:
   a. hold the AM dose of insulin.
   b. administer the AM dose of insulin.
   c. call the physician to report the blood glucose results.
   d. repeat the fingerstick blood glucose test at 0800.

   Rationale: The answer is (b). The fingerstick blood glucose results are within normal limits. The nurse should administer the daily dose of insulin. Options (a), (c), and (d) are not appropriate interventions in this situation.

2. The physician orders isophane NPH insulin 23 units subcut qAM. The nurse carries out this order correctly when the insulin:
   a. dose is given after breakfast.
   b. dose is based on the fingerstick blood glucose results.
   c. is given according to the hospital's qAM schedule.
   d. is administered before breakfast.

   Rationale: The answer is (d). Although daily insulin is ordered qAM, the ordered dose is given before breakfast to correlate with the action of the insulin and food intake. Options (a) and (c) are similar and start after food intake. Option (b) is used mostly with regular insulin.

3. A client with diabetes mellitus type 1 has a correction insulin scale (sliding scale) with regular human insulin listed in the electronic medication record. Based on this finding, it is most important for the nurse to:
   a. administer the regular human insulin on the basis of the fasting blood glucose level.
   b. monitor the client's urine for ketones before meals.
   c. obtain fingerstick blood glucose test before meals.
   d. check the fingerstick blood glucose qid.

   Rationale: The answer is (c). The correction insulin scale (sliding scale) is used to administer regular insulin before meals and at bedtime based on fingerstick blood glucose levels. Options (a), (b), and (d) do not correlate the purpose of the correction insulin scale (sliding scale), regular insulin, blood glucose, and food intake.

1-34 LEGAL CONSIDERATIONS IN NURSING PRACTICE

List the **two types** of **torts**:

1. _____

2. _____

List the **four elements** that constitute **professional negligence:**

1. _____

2. _____

3. _____

4. _____

Draw a line to identify the **unintentional torts.**

Fraud   Invasion of privacy

UNINTENTIONAL TORTS

Assault

Negligence

False imprisonment

Libel

Malpractice

CLINICAL SITUATION   Cassie, a new nursing student, is assigned to Mr. W, a 73-year-old client. Mr. W has kidney disease and has been in the hospital for 3 days. He is alert and wants to know everything about his treatment and questions the nurses all the time. The handoff report indicates that he has had diarrhea all day. He keeps getting out of bed, and the nurses feel that he is getting increasingly weak. Cassie is working with an experienced staff RN. The staff RN instructs Cassie to raise all four bedside rails on Mr. W because she is concerned that he will fall and injure himself.

Pertinent Terminology	Definition
Assault	
Battery	
Libel Slander Negligence Malpractice	
Tort	
Informed Consent	
Standard of Care	

Use the information in the clinical situation to **check off** (✓) the statement or statements below that apply to the situation:

☐ A physician's order is not needed because Mr. W is increasingly weak and the nurse has determined that he is a risk to himself.

☐ The patient's behavior is considered unsafe behavior and bedside rails are not considered restraints.

☐ Raising all four bedside rails would potentially be considered a form of restraint.

☐ It is important to follow the instructions of the experienced RN because she alone is responsible for the care that Mr. W receives.

Collaborative Learning Activity: With a partner, use the clinical situations below to **(1)** check off (✓) the most appropriate action(s) and **(2)** answer the question at the end of the clinical situation.

Clinical Situation	Action(s)
Cindi, a second-year nursing student, has been under a lot of personal stress. She tells another student that she gave her patient the wrong amount of sedative in the morning but that the patient was fine because she carefully monitored his vital signs all day. Cindi is an excellent student and will not allow this to happen again.	☐ The patient was fine—take no action ☐ Fill out an incident/adverse event report ☐ The instructor should be notified ☐ The charge nurse should be notified ☐ The physician should be notified

Cindi **has** or **has not** (*circle one*) been negligent, because _____

_____

Clinical Situation	Action(s)
Mark is a graduate nurse and started working as soon as he received his RN license. He administered medications through the patient's nasogastric tube. During the administration of the medication, the patient began coughing forcefully and gasping for air. Mark noticed that the nasogastric tube had been significantly out of the patient's nose.	☐ Notify the physician ☐ Reinsert tube and listen for placement ☐ Fill out an incident/adverse incident report ☐ Readminister the medications

Mark **has** or **has not** (*circle one*) been negligent, because _____

_____

1-35 REVIEW QUESTIONS

Instructions: Select the most appropriate answer for the following multiple-choice questions.

1. The registered nurse of the medical unit is informed that four clients on the unit have dehydration and diarrhea after eating food contaminated with *Escherichia coli*. Which nursing intervention is most effective in preventing the spread of the organism?
   a. Putting any meat found on the meal tray in the microwave for 2 minutes
   b. Wearing gloves when bathing and assisting the clients
   c. Assigning one nurse to care for the four clients
   d. Washing hands frequently when caring for clients

2. A mother called the clinic nurse to ask whether her son might get head lice because he used a set of earphones 2 days ago that he borrowed from a friend who was just diagnosed with head lice. Which information is most correct to share with the mother? (Select all that apply.)
   a. It is very unlikely that headphones transmit head lice.
   b. Head lice need head-to-head contact to spread.
   c. Use a lice shampoo immediately, even if head lice are not visible.
   d. Adult head lice that lay eggs do not live for more than 24 hours.
   e. Dogs and cats can also transmit head lice.

3. The following vital signs are recorded in the adult client's electronic health record for the day shift: 0800, T 98°F, P 88 (regular), R 24, BP 128/88; 1200, T 99.4°F, P 92 (regular), R 22, BP 124/80. After reviewing the vital signs, which follow-up nursing intervention is most appropriate for the day shift nurse to implement?
   a. Retake the temperature in 1 hour.
   b. Begin cooling measures.
   c. Maintain the client on bed rest until the temperature is normal.
   d. Contact the physician for an antipyretic medication.

4. The nurse is caring for a client who was admitted 2 days ago with hypertension and atrial tachycardia. The handoff report indicates that the client's pulse at 0600 was 122. To apply the assessment phase of the nursing process, it is most important for the nurse to:
   a. ensure that the pulse has been reported to the physician.
   b. plan to monitor the pulse rate q2h.
   c. review the pulse rate for the last 48 hours.
   d. administer the cardiac medications on time.

5. On auscultating the lung sounds of the assigned client, the nurse hears loud vesicular breath sounds on the anterior lateral aspects of the chest during inspiration. The most appropriate follow-up action by the nurse is to:
   a. have the client use the incentive spirometer q1h while awake.
   b. monitor the client for shortness of breath q2h.
   c. check the client's pulse oximetry.
   d. document the findings.

6. The nurse auscultates the abdominal quadrants of a client and immediately hears soft gurgling bowel sounds. Which action by the nurse is most appropriate?
   a. Reassess the bowel sounds in 15 minutes.
   b. Document the findings as assessed.
   c. Record the bowel sounds as "borborygmus."
   d. Ask another nurse to assess the bowel sounds.

7. The nurse is assigned to a patient who has an indwelling urinary catheter and is placed under contact precautions. The patient's plan of care indicates that the patient has methicillin-resistant *Staphylococcus aureus* in the urine. To prevent the spread of infection, it is most important for the nurse to:
   a. wear a mask whenever entering the patient's room.
   b. wear sterile gloves when coming in contact with the patient's urine.
   c. use a gown, gloves, and mask when bathing the patient.
   d. use a gown, gloves, and eye protection to empty the patient's urinary catheter.

8. The nurse is bathing an elderly client at 0800. On turning the client, the nurse finds a small white tablet on the bed. The client takes furosemide (a small white tablet) at 0700 and 1700. It is most appropriate for the nurse to:
   a. record that a small white tablet was found on the client's bed.
   b. administer another dose of furosemide now.
   c. inform the client that the morning dose of furosemide was found on the bed.
   d. recommend that the medications be mixed with soft food to avoid client noncompliance.

9. The physician orders dexamethasone 9 mg direct IV qAM. The nurse finds a vial of dexamethasone 16 mg/mL in the patient's medication drawer. How many mL will the nurse administer to the patient? (Work the problem to the hundredths place and round to the tenths place). Enter your answer:

10. A bird infected with the West Nile virus is bitten by a certain type of mosquito. The virus can then be transmitted to other birds and humans by the mosquito. In this chain of infection, the mosquito is the:
    a. reservoir.
    b. vector.
    c. host.
    d. infectious agent.

11. The nurse writes the following expected outcome in the patient's plan of care for a patient who is diagnosed with a cerebral vascular accident: "The nurse will assist the patient to the chair for meals every day." In applying the nursing process, this expected outcome:
    a. is written appropriately.
    b. is not measurable.
    c. should focus on what the patient can achieve.
    d. should include how long the patient may be in the chair.

12. The nurse is caring for a client who is incontinent of urine. Which nursing intervention is most effective in helping to maintain skin integrity?
    a. Change the incontinence pad q2h and prn.
    b. Limit liquid intake to 1000 mL per day.
    c. Insert an indwelling urinary catheter.
    d. Encourage daily intake of cranberry juice.

13. The nurse receives the following order for a client who is 1 day postop transurethral resection of the prostate: "Irrigate the urinary catheter with NS 0.9% until free of clots." To appropriately implement this order, the nurse would:
    a. instill 100 mL of NS 0.9% every 2 hours into the urinary catheter.
    b. manually irrigate the catheter when clots are visible in the tubing.
    c. clarify the order to include the amount of NS to use.
    d. use clean technique to irrigate the catheter.

14. The nurse is caring for an elderly client just admitted with bronchopneumonia. Which client assessment finding is of greatest concern?
    a. Respirations 26
    b. Bilateral rhonchi
    c. Acute confusion
    d. Yellow-colored sputum

15. The nursing assistant informs the registered nurse that an elderly client, recovering from a cerebral vascular accident, had some difficulty swallowing during breakfast and choked on some food. In monitoring the client for the remainder of the shift, which assessment finding requires immediate follow-up?
    a. Pulse oximetry 98%
    b. 50% oral intake at noon
    c. Pulse 96 at noon; pulse 88 at 0800
    d. Temp 99.6°F at noon; temp 98.6°F at 0800

16. A client had a suprapubic catheter removed 2 days ago and is now being discharged. What is most important for the nurse to include in the discharge teaching?
    a. Urinary incontinence is normal for 1 to 2 weeks.
    b. Practice Kegel exercises five times per day.
    c. Empty the bladder every 2 to 3 hours for the first week.
    d. Limit fluid intake for the first week.

17. The nurse is delegating the care of a client who is 1 day postop to the nursing assistant. The nursing assistant asks whether the client's sequential stockings can be removed during the bath. Which response is most appropriate?
    a. "Do not remove the sequential stockings until tomorrow."
    b. "The sequential stockings can be removed while bathing the client."
    c. "Turn off the compression control device, but do not remove the sequential stockings."
    d. "Remove the sequential stocking as you begin to wash each leg, but reapply it immediately."

18. A 55-year-old female patient is diagnosed with stress incontinence. The nurse is most correct to prepare to:
    a. instruct the patient regarding the need to decrease fluid intake.
    b. provide the patient with adult incontinence pads.
    c. provide information regarding Kegel exercises.
    d. help the patient recognize emotionally stressful situations that contribute to incontinence.

19. The nurse is reading the plan of care of a patient and notices that the expected outcome was for the patient to eat 90% of the regular diet by today. The handoff report indicates that the patient has been eating 50% of each meal for the last 24 hours. Which action by the nurse is most appropriate initially?
    a. Request the family bring in foods that the patient likes.
    b. Assess the current needs of the patient.
    c. Provide the patient with between-meal snacks.
    d. Validate that the documentation in the EMR is correct.

20. In the handoff report, the nurse learns that the assigned client has a Cheyne-Stokes breathing pattern. Which of the following would the nurse expect to see? (Select all that apply.)
    a. Periods of apnea
    b. Deep, rapid breathing
    c. Shallow breathing
    d. Respiratory rate of 12 or less
    e. Full inspiration and expiration

21. The nurse is assigned to a client who receives furosemide 40 mg IVP q12h and digoxin 0.25 mg po qAM. To administer the morning dose of these drugs safely, the nurse should do which of the following? (Select all that apply.)
    a. Hold the digoxin if there are complaints of blurred vision.
    b. Monitor for signs of increased serum Na$^+$ level.
    c. Hold the drugs if diuresis noted.
    d. Monitor for symptoms of decreased serum K$^+$ level.
    e. Take the apical pulse for 30 seconds and multiply by 2.

22. A client is 4 days postop right total hip replacement with a cemented prosthesis. To prevent right hip dislocation, it is important to tell the client which of the following? (Select all that apply.)
    a. Bend at the waist to pick up items.
    b. Do not apply any weight on the right leg.
    c. Use an elevated toilet seat.
    d. Do not cross legs.
    e. Avoid lying on the right hip.

23. The nurse is caring for a client who is 3 days postop abdominal surgery. On changing the abdominal dressing, the nurse notes the surgical incision has eviscerated. The nurse is correct in doing which of the following? (Select all that apply.)
    a. Keep the client on bed rest.
    b. Apply a dry sterile dressing on the wound.
    c. Monitor vital signs q2h.
    d. Place a moist sterile dressing on the wound.
    e. Encourage fluid intake.

24. The nurse is assigned to care for a client diagnosed with diabetes mellitus type 1. The physician orders glargine insulin 22 units qPM, fingerstick blood glucose testing AC and at bedtime, and a correction insulin scale (sliding scale) with regular human insulin. To appropriately implement the correction insulin order, the nurse will plan to administer the regular human insulin (Select all that apply.):
    a. every time the fingerstick blood glucose is tested.
    b. on the basis of the fingerstick blood glucose results.
    c. 30 minutes after each meal and at bedtime.
    d. in combination with the glargine insulin PM dose.
    e. 5 units before each meal and bedtime.

25. The nurse admits an adult client diagnosed with a bowel obstruction. The physician orders the following: (1) NPO and (2) insert a nasogastric tube to low wall suction. To implement the orders, the nurse would do which of the following? (Select all that apply.)
    a. Use a 10 F nasogastric tube.
    b. Use a 14 F nasogastric tube.
    c. Provide the client with water during insertion of the nasogastric tube.
    d. Manually aspirate all gastric contents immediately after nasogastric tube insertion.
    e. Ensure that the nasogastric tube is connected to the suction equipment before inserting the tube.

Priority Setting and Decision Making

2-1 STANDARDS OF PROFESSIONAL PERFORMANCE

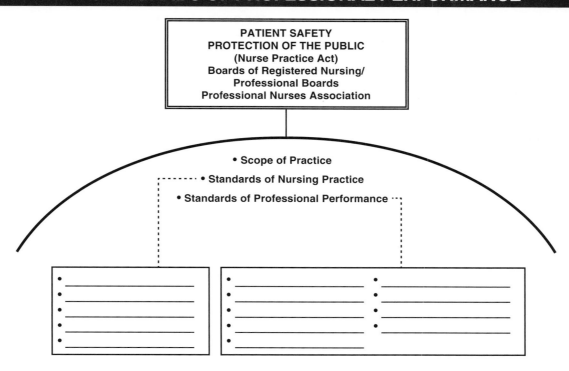

```
PATIENT SAFETY
PROTECTION OF THE PUBLIC
(Nurse Practice Act)
Boards of Registered Nursing/
Professional Boards
Professional Nurses Association
```

- Scope of Practice
- Standards of Nursing Practice
- Standards of Professional Performance

CLINICAL SITUATION The RN on the medical-surgical unit has been a staff member for 15 years. She is clinically very competent and establishes good rapport with clients and their families. The RN has currently been assigned to work with nursing students. Several of the students have complained that it is difficult to work with this RN because she prefers to work independently and rarely answers the students' questions. The RN has commented to other staff that she only agreed to take students because the supervisor wants nursing students on the unit.

Pertinent Terminology	Definition
American Nurses Association (ANA) Canadian Nurses Association (CNA)	
Standards of Nursing Practice	
Standards of Professional Performance	

- Use the ANA Standards of Professional Performance to identify the behaviors that represent professional performance.
- Using the clinical situation, put an **"X"** in the middle column to identify the staff RN's professional performance behaviors that need strengthening.

ANA Standards of Professional Performance		Write in behaviors that describe professional performance for each standard.
Quality of Practice		
Education		
Practice Evaluation		
Collegiality		
Collaboration		
Ethics		
Research		
Resource Utilization		
Leadership		

Collaborative Learning Activity: With a partner, discuss the following statements related to "standards." <u>Underline</u> the statements that are **TRUE.**

1. Standards, such as the Standards of Nursing Practice and Standards of Professional Practice, are considered legally binding regulations.

2. Standards of Nursing Practice can be used in a court of law in malpractice cases.

3. Standards of Nursing Practice identify the minimal expectations in the delivery of nursing care.

4. Professional nurses working in the outpatient setting are not held to the same standards of nursing practice as are professional nurses working in the acute care setting.

5. Additional standards of nursing care may be required in specialty areas such as medical-surgical units, pediatric units, and critical care units.

2-2 THE PATIENT UNDERGOING SURGERY

0700 Handoff Report:

S	Mr. H, age 60, was admitted for persistent abdominal pain. He is diagnosed with gastric cancer and is scheduled for a partial gastrectomy later this morning. Mr. H is very anxious after speaking with his wife and indicates that he will not sign the surgical consent. He just told me that he is having abdominal pain and "wants his pain shot right now." He has an NPO order starting at 0800.
B	He states he has had nausea and vomiting and has noticed a 10-lb weight loss within the last 2 months.
A	He has an intact and patent IV of 0.9% sodium chloride at 125 mL/hr in the right forearm. He has morphine sulfate 10 mg q3h IV prn five ondansetron hydrochloride 4 mg IV q8h prn nausea, and aluminum hydroxide 30 mL po q2h prn abdominal pain. It is just about 3 hours since his last pain medication and the aluminum hydroxide was given 2 hours ago. Baseline vital signs are: T 98.8°F, P 98, R 20, B/P 148/92, pulse ox 96%, pain level 7.
R	The following nursing interventions are recommended:

Prioritize the following five **recommended nursing interventions** as you, the nurse, would do them to initially take care of Mr. H. Write a number in the box to identify the order of your interventions (#1 = first intervention, #2 = second intervention, etc.), and state a **rationale** for each intervention.

INTERVENTIONS	PRIORITY #	RATIONALE
• Administer IV pain med	☐	_____
• Sit and talk with patient	☐	_____
• Give aluminum hydroxide 30 mL	☐	_____
• Offer to call a family member	☐	_____
• Notify physician	☐	_____

KEY POINTS TO CONSIDER _____

Mr. H does consent to have surgery and returns to the medical unit postoperatively. He has an IV of lactated Ringer's solution infusing at 125 mL/hr and you assess the following:
1. P 90, R 20, BP 130/76, pulse ox 94%, pain level 2
2. He is alert and oriented and his skin is warm and dry
3. NG tube draining brown reddish drainage (300 mL in the last 4 hours)
4. Indwelling urinary catheter draining light yellow urine (700 mL in the last 4 hours)
5. Abdominal dressing intact and dry

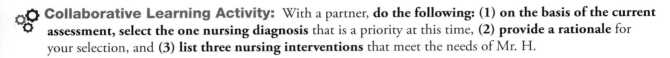 **Collaborative Learning Activity:** With a partner, **do the following: (1) on the basis of the current assessment, select the one nursing diagnosis** that is a priority at this time, **(2) provide a rationale** for your selection, and **(3) list three nursing interventions** that meet the needs of Mr. H.

All of the following nursing diagnoses may apply to Mr. H:

Risk for infection, Acute pain, Anxiety, Ineffective airway clearance, Fatigue, Impaired physical mobility, Imbalanced nutrition: less than body requirements, Deficient knowledge, Risk for deficient fluid volume, Fear

Nursing Diagnosis	Rationale	Nursing Interventions

Several hours after surgery you note that Mr. H is very restless and you assess:

R 32, P 130, BP 108/70, pulse ox 90%, NG drainage 200 mL bright red drainage, skin cool, c/o a dull constant pain in the abdomen with a pain level of 8

Based on the situation, identify and write the **priority problem** in the box below. Then, starting with the small box labeled **#1, prioritize** the **nursing interventions** for this situation and identify your plan for follow-up care for Mr. H.

NURSING INTERVENTIONS

A. Monitor P, R, BP, and pulse oximetry

B. Record assessment/nursing care

C. Assess LOC and neuro status

D. Plan to start oxygen therapy

E. Stay with Mr. H

F. Notify physician

DECISION-MAKING DIAGRAM

New Action Plan

#1   #2   #3   #4   #5   #6

Priority Problem

NOTES _____

_____

APPLYING CRITICAL THINKING SKILLS TO TEST QUESTIONS

INSTRUCTIONS: Circle the one best answer for each test question. Write your rationale for selecting the answer. To enhance your learning and test-taking skills, discuss your answer and rationale with a partner. The answer and the rationale can be found on the back of this page.

1. The nurse assesses the following on a client who had a colon resection 5 days ago: A & O ×4, skin warm, abdomen distended nontender, bowel sounds present. Abdominal sutures well approximated. States pain level 2 out of 10 on the pain scale. Fine crackles in the bilateral lower lung bases. In planning care, which nursing action is of priority?
   a. Take vital signs q4h.
   b. Ambulate the client.
   c. Assess lung sounds q4h.
   d. Push oral fluids.

   Rationale for your selection: _____
   _____
   _____
   _____
   _____

2. The nurse is caring for a client who has diabetes mellitus type 1. The client takes clopidrogrel (Plavix) 75 mg po daily and aspirin 81 mg po daily. In preparing the administration of these drugs, it is most important for the nurse to first
   a. assess whether the client is having mild pain.
   b. check the serum prothrombin time levels.
   c. monitor the blood pressure.
   d. ensure that the client has eaten.

   Rationale for your selection: _____
   _____
   _____
   _____
   _____

3. A patient is complaining of right lower quadrant abdominal pain. In assessing the abdomen of the patient, the nurse is most accurate to begin by
   a. palpating the right lower quadrant first.
   b. auscultating the upper abdominal quadrants first and then the lower abdominal quadrants.
   c. percussing gently starting from the top of the abdomen and comparing from left to right.
   d. inspecting the contour of the abdomen.

   Rationale for your selection: _____
   _____
   _____
   _____
   _____
   _____

ANSWER KEY FOR
APPLYING CRITICAL THINKING SKILLS TO TEST QUESTIONS

HELPFUL HINTS: Read all test questions carefully. Identify key words in the question that will guide you in answering the question. In these test questions the **key words** to consider are **"priority," "most important,"** and **"most appropriate."** Compare your rationale with the one in the test question.

1. The nurse assesses the following on a client who had a colon resection 5 days ago: A & O ×4, skin warm, abdomen distended nontender, bowel sounds present. Abdominal sutures well approximated. States pain level 2 out of 10 on the pain scale. Fine crackles in the bilateral lower lung bases. In planning care, which nursing action is of priority?
   a. Take vital signs q4h.
   (b.) Ambulate the client.
   c. Assess lung sounds q4h.
   d. Push oral fluids.

   Rationale: The answer is (b). Assessment data indicate the need to ambulate the client to ease abdominal distention and enhance respiration and movement of secretions. Options (a), (c), and (d) are important but do not help the client with the priority problems.

2. The nurse is caring for a client who has diabetes mellitus type 1. The client takes clopidrogrel (Plavix) 75 mg po daily and aspirin 81 mg po daily. In preparing the administration of these drugs, it is most important for the nurse to first
   a. assess whether the client is having mild pain.
   (b.) check the serum prothrombin time levels.
   c. monitor the blood pressure.
   d. ensure that the client has eaten.

   Rationale: The answer is (b). Clopidogrel and aspirin both have anticoagulation properties. Coagulation studies should be monitored throughout therapy. Options (a), (c), and (d) do not address the most important intervention related to this drug therapy.

3. A patient is complaining of right lower quadrant abdominal pain. In assessing the abdomen of the patient, the nurse is most accurate to begin by
   a. palpating the right lower quadrant first.
   b. auscultating the upper abdominal quadrants first and then the lower abdominal quadrants.
   c. percussing gently starting from the top of the abdomen and comparing from left to right.
   (d.) inspecting the contour of the abdomen.

   Rationale: The answer is (d). Abdominal assessment begins with inspection followed by auscultation, palpation, and percussion. Options (a), (b), and (c) should be performed after inspection, in the following order: auscultation, palpation, percussion.

2-3 THE PATIENT WITH AN INTESTINAL OBSTRUCTION

0700 Handoff Report:

S	Mrs. W, 56 years old, is hospitalized with the diagnosis of small bowel obstruction. She has an NG tube to low continuous suction draining dark brown drainage. The nursing assistant just reported that Mrs. W just vomited 100 mL of dark brown secretions.
B	Mrs. W experienced constant vomiting prior to coming to the ER last night. She received an antiemetic in the ER and came to our unit around 3 AM.
A	IV of D5/0.45% NaCl with 30 mEq potassium chloride (KCl) infusing at 100 mL/hr. Her skin is warm and dry and her mucous membranes are dry. Her abdomen is distended with hyperactive bowel sounds in the right upper and lower quadrants.
R	The following nursing interventions are recommended:

2 Priority Setting and Decision Making

Prioritize the following five **recommended nursing interventions** as you would do them to initially take care of Mrs. W. Write a number in the box to identify the order of your interventions (#1 = first intervention, #2 = second intervention, etc.), and state a **rationale** for each intervention.

INTERVENTIONS	PRIORITY #	RATIONALE
• Provide thorough mouth care	☐	_____
• Assess abdomen, measure abdominal girth	☐	_____
• Assess NG tube and suction	☐	_____
• Take the vital signs	☐	_____
⚠ • Ensure Mrs. W is in semi-Fowler's position	☐	_____

KEY POINTS TO CONSIDER _____

_____

_____

After 48 hours Mrs. W's abdomen is less distended and the current assessment findings include:
1. Hemoglobin 9.2 g, hematocrit 29%, K^+ 3.1 mEq, Na^+ 145 mEq
2. T 98.8°F, P 92, irregular, R 20, BP 152/94, pulse ox 94%
3. NG tube draining dark brown drainage (250 mL in the last 8 hours)
4. Pain on a scale of 1 to 10 = 4
5. No stool or passing of flatus, urine output last 24 hours 600 mL

Collaborative Learning Activity: With a partner, **do the following: (1) based on the current assessment, select the one nursing diagnosis** that is a priority at this time, **(2) provide a rationale** for your selection, and **(3) list three nursing interventions** that meet the needs of Mrs. W.

All of the following nursing diagnoses may apply to Mrs. W:

Risk for infection, Acute pain, Anxiety, Ineffective airway clearance, Imbalanced nutrition: less than body requirements, Deficient knowledge, Deficient fluid volume, Risk for impaired skin integrity, Fear, Disturbed sleep pattern

Nursing Diagnosis	Rationale	Nursing Interventions

The next day, Mrs. W's assessment included the following: NG output 500 mL and urine output 100 mL dark amber during the night shift. Faint bowel sounds, capillary refill greater than 5 seconds. Weak, lethargic, and disoriented. Mucous membranes dry. Orthostatic BP 148/90 (lying), 124/84 (sitting).

On the basis of the situation, identify and write the **priority problem** in the box below. Then, starting with the small box labeled **#1, prioritize** the **nursing interventions** for this situation and identify your follow-up action plan for Mrs. W.

NURSING INTERVENTIONS

A. Monitor IV fluid replacement

B. Inform physician

C. Orient Mrs. W

D. Provide oral care

E. Raise side rails

F. Take vital signs

DECISION-MAKING DIAGRAM

New Action Plan

#1 #2 #3 #4 #5 #6

Priority Problem

NOTES _____

_____

APPLYING CRITICAL THINKING SKILLS TO TEST QUESTIONS

INSTRUCTIONS: Circle the one best answer for each test question. Write your rationale for selecting the answer. To enhance your learning and test-taking skills, discuss your answer and rationale with a partner. The answer and the rationale can be found on the back of this page.

2 Priority Setting and Decision Making

1. The nurse is taking care of a client who has an NG tube to continuous low suction. The nursing assistant reports that the client has vomited 100 mL of light yellow greenish fluid. It is most important for the nurse to initially
   a. check the medication record for an antiemetic.
   b. check NG tube placement.
   c. add the emesis to the total output for the shift.
   d. ask the client whether the desire to vomit has decreased.

   Rationale for your selection: _____
   _____
   _____
   _____

2. The health care provider ordered the patient's nasogastric (NG) tube to be removed this morning. To implement this order the registered nurse (Select all that apply)
   a. should measure the NG tube output for the shift.
   b. may delegate the NG tube removal to the LVN/LPN.
   c. uses sterile technique to remove the NG tube.
   d. assists the patient to a semi-Fowler's position.
   e. instructs the patient to hold his or her breath during removal.

   Rationale for your selection: _____
   _____
   _____
   _____

3. The client is receiving continuous full-strength formula tube feeding through an NG feeding tube at 75 mL/hr, and there are 100 mL left in the feeding bag. The nurse is preparing to administer the 0900 furosemide 10 mg tablet. Which technique demonstrates safety in the administration of the medication?
   a. Crush the medication, dissolve in water, and put in the feeding bag.
   b. Stop the formula tube feeding for 15 min prior to administering the medication.
   c. Check tube placement prior to administering the medication.
   d. Crush the medication, dissolve in water, and administer directly into feeding tube.

   Rationale for your selection: _____
   _____
   _____
   _____

ANSWER KEY FOR
APPLYING CRITICAL THINKING SKILLS TO TEST QUESTIONS

HELPFUL HINTS: Read all test questions carefully. Identify key words in the question that will guide you in answering the question. In these test questions the **key words** to consider are **"most important"** and **"safety."** Compare your rationale with the one found for each question.

1. The nurse is taking care of a client who has an NG tube to continuous low suction. The nursing assistant reports that the client has vomited 100 mL of light yellow greenish fluid. It is most important for the nurse to initially
   a. check the medication record for an antiemetic.
   b. check NG tube placement.
   c. add the emesis to the total output for the shift.
   d. ask the client whether the desire to vomit has decreased.

   Rationale: The answer is (b). Vomiting should not be experienced with the use of an NG tube. Tube placement should be assessed. Option (a) is not the initial intervention, and options (c) and (d) are not the most important interventions.

2. The health care provider ordered the patient's nasogastric (NG) tube to be removed this morning. To implement this order the registered nurse (Select all that apply)
   a. should measure the NG tube output for the shift.
   b. may delegate the NG tube removal to the LVN/LPN.
   c. uses sterile technique to remove the NG tube.
   d. assists the patient to a semi-Fowler's position.
   e. instructs the patient to hold his or her breath during removal.

   Rationale: The answer is (a, b, d, e). This procedure may be delegated to the LVN/LPN. Placing the patient in a semi-Fowler's position ensures comfort and safety, and having the patient hold his or her breath closes the epiglottis and helps prevent fluid from the tube from entering into the lungs. Measuring output helps with appropriate documentation. Option (c), NG tube removal, is not a sterile procedure.

3. The client is receiving continuous full-strength formula tube feeding through an NG feeding tube at 75 mL/hr and there are 100 mL left in the feeding bag. The nurse is preparing to administer the 0900 furosemide 10 mg tablet. Which technique demonstrates safety in the administration of the medication?
   a. Crush the medications, dissolve in water, and put in the feeding bag.
   b. Stop the formula tube feeding for 15 min prior to administering the medication.
   c. Check tube placement prior to administering the medication.
   d. Crush the medications, dissolve in water, and administer directly into feeding tube.

   Rationale: The answer is (c). Tube placement should be checked before administration of medication or formula feeding. Options (a), (b), and (d) do not describe the technique that addresses safety.

2-4 THE PATIENT WITH A COLOSTOMY

1500 Handoff Report:

S	Mrs. P, 42 years old, had surgery today for colon cancer. She had a sigmoid colostomy this morning. She was transferred to her room 2 hours ago. She is sleeping but arouses easily. She needs to be reminded to use the PCA. There is an order for her to sit at the side of the bed this evening. The morning laboratory work includes a CBC.
B	The history and physical indicate that Mrs. P is worried that the surgery will not remove all of the cancer.
A	Her latest VS: T 98°F, P 86, R 18, BP 132/88, pain level 3 out of 10 on the pain scale. Sequential stockings are on. She has a colostomy bag in place with the stoma edematous and red. The surgical dressing is clean and dry. The NG tube is to low continuous wall suction draining dark brown drainage. She has a right double-lumen central line with total parenteral nutrition (TPN) infusing at 83 mL/hr, and an IV of D5/0.9% NaCl with a PCA (morphine sulfate) set to deliver 1 mg/6 min per patient demand, not to exceed 30 mg in 4 hours.
R	The follow-up assessment interventions are recommended:

Prioritize the following five **recommended nursing interventions** as you, the nurse, would do them to initially take care of Mrs. P. Write a number in the box to identify the order of your interventions (#1 = first intervention, #2 = second intervention, etc.), and state a **rationale** for each intervention.

INTERVENTIONS	PRIORITY #	RATIONALE
• Assess surgical dressing and stoma	☐	_____
• Take the vital signs	☐	_____
• Assess pain level	☐	_____
• Check NG tube and drainage	☐	_____
• Check IV site, TPN, and PCA setting	☐	_____

KEY POINTS TO CONSIDER _____
_____
_____
_____

(sidebar) **2** Priority Setting and Decision Making

The **first postop day** assessment was significant for the following signs and symptoms:
1. Bowel sounds absent
2. Mrs. P moans when she turns in bed
3. Weak, ineffective cough
4. Stoma swollen and reddened

⚙ **Collaborative Learning Activity:** With a partner, **do the following: (1) select the one nursing diagnosis** that is a priority at this time, **(2) provide a rationale** for your selection, and **(3) list three nursing interventions** that assist you to meet the needs of the patient.

All of the following nursing diagnoses may apply to Mrs. P:

Risk for infection, Risk for impaired skin integrity, Acute pain, Anxiety, Ineffective airway clearance, Fatigue, Delayed surgical recovery, Imbalanced nutrition: less than body requirements, Disturbed body image, Risk for deficient fluid volume, Fear

Nursing Diagnosis	Rationale	Nursing Interventions

On the morning of the **third postop day,** the NG tube was removed per the physician's order, and Mrs. P was started on a clear liquid diet. In the afternoon the assessment findings included: stoma edematous and dusky, abdomen distended, pain level 8 out of 10 on the pain scale.

On the basis of the **third postop day** assessment, identify and write the **priority problem** in the box below. Then, starting with the small box labeled **#1, prioritize** the **nursing interventions** listed and **identify** your action plan for the follow-up care of Mrs. P.

NURSING INTERVENTIONS　　　　**DECISION-MAKING DIAGRAM**

A. Take the vital signs

B. Prepare to insert NG tube

C. Assess colostomy bag and bowel sounds

D. Notify physician stat

E. Place on NPO

F. Check IV patency

New Action Plan

#1　#2　#3　#4　#5　#6

Priority Problem

NOTES _____

APPLYING CRITICAL THINKING SKILLS TO TEST QUESTIONS

INSTRUCTIONS: Circle the one best answer for each test question. Write your rationale for selecting the answer. To enhance your learning and test-taking skills, discuss your answer and rationale with a partner. The answer and the rationale can be found on the back of this page.

1. The handoff report of a client indicates that a double-barrel colostomy was performed 2 days ago. Which assessment finding is of most concern?
   a. Right-sided colostomy bag with small amount fecal drainage, left-sided colostomy bag with serosanguineous mucous drainage
   b. Right-sided colostomy bag with serosanguineous mucous drainage. Stoma dark red. Left-sided colostomy bag with minimal drainage
   c. Abdomen soft, tender to touch, stoma red and edematous
   d. Bowel sounds hypoactive on right side; absent on left side

   Rationale for your selection: _____
   _____
   _____
   _____

2. The nurse is assigned to a client who was had an ileostomy 3 days ago and is now started on a clear liquid diet. The client is receiving IV fluid set at 75 mL/hr. Which of the following interventions is most important for the nurse to ask the nursing assistant to perform?
   a. Take vital signs q4h.
   b. Monitor intake and output q8h.
   c. Give 500 mL of fluids for the shift.
   d. Assist the client to turn in bed q4h.

   Rationale for your selection: _____
   _____
   _____
   _____

3. The client is 72 years old and is admitted with a respiratory tract infection. The client is on erythromycin 400 mg q6h po. The client has a sigmoid colostomy. Which of the following assessment findings would be most indicative of a potential complication?
   a. Admission white blood cell count of 11,500
   b. Six liquid stools during the shift
   c. T 100.8°F during morning assessment
   d. Urinary output of 260 mL for the last 4 hours

   Rationale for your selection: _____
   _____
   _____
   _____

ANSWER KEY FOR
APPLYING CRITICAL THINKING SKILLS TO TEST QUESTIONS

HELPFUL HINTS: Read all test questions carefully. Identify key words in the question that will guide you in answering the question. In these test questions the **key words** to consider are **"most concern," "most important,"** and **"most indicative."** Compare your rationale with the one found for each question.

1. The handoff report of a client indicates that a double-barrel colostomy was performed 2 days ago. Which assessment finding is of most concern?
   a. Right-sided colostomy bag with small amount fecal drainage, left-sided colostomy bag with serosanguineous mucous drainage
   b. Right-sided colostomy bag with serosanguineous mucous drainage. Stoma dark red. Left-sided colostomy bag with minimal drainage
   c. Abdomen soft, tender to touch, stoma red and edematous
   d. Bowel sounds hypoactive on right side; absent on left side

Rationale: The answer is (b). The dark red color of the stoma is an indication of possible impaired perfusion of the stoma. Options (a), (c), and (d) are normal assessment findings consistent with the situation.

2. The nurse is assigned to a client who was had an ileostomy 3 days ago and is now started on a clear liquid diet. The client is receiving IV fluid set at 75 mL/hr. Which of the following interventions is most important for the nurse to ask the nursing assistant to perform?
   a. Take vital signs q4h.
   b. Monitor intake and output q8h.
   c. Give 500 mL of fluids for the shift.
   d. Assist the client to turn in bed q4h.

Rationale: The answer is (c). A new ileostomy will initially drain up to 2 L/day. Replacing fluid to prevent dehydration is important. Options (a), (b), and (d) are good interventions, but the client needs hydration because of the fluid loss.

3. The client is 72 years old and is admitted with a respiratory tract infection. The client is on erythromycin 400 mg q6h po. The client has a sigmoid colostomy. Which of the following assessment findings would be most indicative of a potential complication?
   a. Admission white blood cell count of 11,500
   b. Six liquid stools during the shift
   c. T 100.8°F during morning assessment
   d. Urinary output of 260 mL for the last 4 hours

Rationale: The answer is (b). Erythromycin can cause diarrhea. With a sigmoid colostomy the client should have near-to-normal stools. Options (a) and (c) are symptoms associated with an infection, for which the client was admitted. Option (d) is within normal limits.

2-5 THE PATIENT WITH COLON CANCER

0800 Handoff Report:

S	Mr. S, 65 years old, has colon cancer. He is admitted for a colon resection. In preparation for surgery, his current orders include NPO, insert an NG tube, and a saline lock. He is to receive his preop medication at 12:00 pm today.
B	His current medical history is significant for complaints of changes in bowel habits/constipation, passing of bloody stools, abdominal pain, and weight loss. His past medical condition includes a history of coronary artery disease and hypertension. In addition to antihypertensive medication, he was taking aspirin 81 mg po daily. He states he stopped the aspirin 3 days ago as recommend by his physician.
A	His 6:00 AM vital signs are T 98°F, P 78, R 20, BP 162/90, pulse ox 95%, pain level 3, states that it feels like "abdominal cramping."
R	The following nursing interventions are recommended:

Prioritize the five **recommended nursing interventions** as you, the nurse, would do them to initially take care of Mr. S. Write a number in the box to identify the order of your interventions (#1 = first intervention, #2 = second intervention, etc.), and state a **rationale** for each intervention.

INTERVENTIONS	PRIORITY #	RATIONALE
• Perform a body systems	☐	_____
• Take the vital signs	☐	_____
• Insert saline lock	☐	_____
• Insert NG tube	☐	_____
• Check surgical consent	☐	_____

KEY POINTS TO CONSIDER _____

_____

_____

_____

A colon resection is done on Mr. S. The **first postop day** assessment includes:
1. Lactated Ringer's infusing at 100 mL/hr and PCA with morphine sulfate
2. Elastic stockings on; intermittent compression device ordered for 24 hours
3. NG tube to low continuous wall suction draining brown greenish fluid
4. Wants to stay in a low Fowler's position
5. Short and shallow respirations

Collaborative Learning Activity: With a partner, **do the following: (1)** based on the **first postop day assessment, select the one nursing diagnosis** that is a priority at this time, **(2) provide a rationale** for your selection, and **(3) list three nursing interventions** that meet the needs of Mr. S.

All of the following nursing diagnoses may apply to Mr. S:

Risk for infection, Acute pain, Anxiety, Ineffective airway clearance, Imbalanced nutrition: less than body requirements, Deficient knowledge, Risk for deficient fluid volume, Risk for impaired skin integrity, Risk for ineffective peripheral tissue perfusion, Fear

Nursing Diagnosis	Rationale	Nursing Interventions

On the **fourth postoperative day,** you assess the following signs and symptoms on Mr. S:

- Complaints of tenderness in the right calf with a positive Homans' sign
- 2+ right ankle/calf edema; no edema noted on left ankle/calf
- Right calf is warmer to touch than the left calf

Based on the **fourth postoperative day** assessment, identify and write the **priority problem** in the box below. Then, starting with the small box labeled **#1, prioritize** the **nursing interventions** listed and **identify** your action plan for the follow-up care of Mr. S.

NURSING INTERVENTIONS   **DECISION-MAKING DIAGRAM**

A. Elevate right extremity

B. Notify physician

C. Maintain bed rest   **New Action Plan**
                                        #1   #2   #3   #4   #5   #6

D. Allay Mr. S's concerns

E. Administer mild analgesic if
   ordered

                                        Priority Problem   **NOTES** _____

F. Assess pedal pulses

APPLYING CRITICAL THINKING SKILLS TO TEST QUESTIONS

INSTRUCTIONS: Circle the one best answer for each test question. Write your rationale for selecting the answer. To enhance your learning and test-taking skills, discuss your answer and rationale with a partner. The answer and the rationale can be found on the back of this page.

1. The nurse is caring for a client who had an ileostomy 5 days ago. The ileostomy is draining large amounts of green brownish liquid stool. On discharge, the client asks the nurse whether the stool consistency will eventually become more solid. Which response by the nurse is best?
   a. "The stool will become solid as the ileostomy heals."
   b. "Eating certain foods can help make the stool more solid."
   c. "It takes about 1 year to see exactly what the stool consistency will be."
   d. "The stool will change to a mushy consistency after several months."

   Rationale for your selection: _____
   _____
   _____
   _____

2. The nurse is providing discharge instructions to a client who is going home after having an ileostomy for colon cancer. A priority discharge instruction is to instruct the client to
   a. irrigate the ileostomy weekly.
   b. drink eight glasses of water daily.
   c. monitor the daily output from the ileostomy.
   d. use a mild laxative if there is no ileostomy drainage for 24 hours.

   Rationale for your selection: _____
   _____
   _____
   _____

3. The nurse is assisting a client to irrigate his colostomy. After instilling the water, the client has no output. What should the nurse do next?
   a. Encourage the client to ambulate.
   b. Irrigate the colostomy again within 30 minutes.
   c. Digitally stimulate the colostomy opening.
   d. Notify the physician.

   Rationale for your selection: _____
   _____
   _____
   _____

ANSWER KEY FOR
APPLYING CRITICAL THINKING SKILLS TO TEST QUESTIONS

HELPFUL HINTS: Read all test questions carefully. Identify key words in the question that will guide you in answering the question. In these test questions the **key words** to consider are **"best," "priority,"** and **"next."** Compare your rationale with the one in the test question.

1. The nurse is caring for a client who had an ileostomy 5 days ago. The ileostomy is draining large amounts of green brownish liquid stool. On discharge, the client asks the nurse whether the stool consistency will eventually become more solid. Which response by the nurse is best?
   a. "The stool will become solid as the ileostomy heals."
   b. "Eating certain foods can help make the stool more solid."
   c. "It takes about 1 year to see exactly what the stool consistency will be."
   ⓓ "The stool will change to a mushy consistency after several months."

Rationale: The answer is (d). Fecal drainage from an ileostomy is mostly liquid and changes to a mushy consistency in 3 to 6 months. Options (a), (b), and (c) do not provide the client with the correct information.

2. The nurse is providing discharge instructions to a client who is going home after having an ileostomy for colon cancer. A priority discharge instruction is to instruct the client to
   a. irrigate the ileostomy weekly.
   ⓑ drink eight glasses of water daily.
   c. monitor the daily output from the ileostomy.
   d. use a mild laxative if there is no ileostomy drainage for 24 hours.

Rationale: The answer is (b). Daily fecal drainage from a new ileostomy can range from 1000 to 2000 mL. The client is at risk for dehydration along with fluid and electrolyte imbalance. Options (a) and (d) are interventions that do not apply to the care of an ileostomy. Option (c) is good but does not help the client prevent a complication.

3. The nurse is assisting a client to irrigate his colostomy. After instilling the water, the client has no output. What should the nurse do next?
   ⓐ Encourage the client to ambulate.
   b. Irrigate the colostomy again within 30 minutes.
   c. Digitally stimulate the colostomy opening.
   d. Notify the physician.

Rationale: The answer is (a). Ambulation can stimulate peristalsis and the flow of fecal drainage. Option (b) would instill more fluid and may cause trauma and excessive loss of fluid and electrolytes. Option (c) is not appropriate, and option (d) is not necessary because it may take some time for the drainage to begin.

2-6 THE PATIENT WITH TOTAL PARENTERAL NUTRITION

0800 Handoff Report:

 In the handoff report you learn that your patient, Mrs. FJM, is improving. She had only 1 watery stool during the night shift. The 0600 vital signs are: T 98.8°F, P 76, R 18, BP 140/94, pulse ox 95%. At 0600, she complained of pain in her right lower leg at a pain level of 3, the patient said it feels like an achy dull feeling that was present when she awoke. No edema noted, pedal pulse is present. Blood glucose was done.

The following patient care plan information is available:

VS q4h I & O (✓) Weigh qAM BRP with assist prn Admit date: 3/16 Name: FJM Age: 55	℞ subclavian central line inserted 3/16 Parenteral nutrition (PN) per IV pump @ 83 mL/hr Lipids 10% (M-W-F) infuse over 12 hours BG fingersticks q6h (6-12-6-12) Dx: Dehydration/Diarrhea Hx of Crohn's disease with acute exacerbation, atrial fibrillation, smoker, 1 pack per week	Diet: NPO Routine med: Vit. K 10 mg subcut qMon Regular insulin 2 units if BG = 180–200 mg/dL Call MD if BG more than 200 mg/dL

Prioritize the following five **recommended nursing interventions** as you would do them to take care of Mrs. FJM. Write a number in the box to identify the order of your interventions (#1 = first intervention, #2 = second intervention, etc.), and state a **rationale** for each intervention.

INTERVENTIONS	PRIORITY #	RATIONALE
• Perform a body systems physical assessment	☐	_____
• Assess right leg	☐	_____
• Assess central line for patency and central line dressing	☐	_____
• Get 0600 blood glucose results	☐	_____
• Assess right arm and neck for distention	☐	_____

KEY POINTS TO CONSIDER _____
_____
_____

Priority Setting and Decision Making — **2**

Mrs. FJM was taken to x-ray 1 hour ago. On her return to the unit, the IV pump is beeping and you are informed that the machine has been beeping for a long time. You assess the following:
1. PN not infusing
2. Skin warm, diaphoretic, complains of nervousness and rapid heartbeat
3. VS: T 98°F, P 118, R 26, BP 136/90, pulse ox 96%, right lower leg pain level 4, dull achy pain

⚙ **Collaborative Learning Activity:** With a partner, **do the following: (1) select the one nursing diagnosis** that is a priority at this time, **(2) provide a rationale** for your selection, and **(3) list the nursing interventions** that assist you to meet the needs of the patient.

All of the following nursing diagnoses may apply to Mrs. FJM:

Anxiety, Risk for infection, Risk for activity intolerance, Risk for imbalanced fluid volume, Impaired tissue integrity, Ineffective peripheral tissue perfusion, Imbalanced nutrition: less than body requirements, Risk for unstable blood glucose level, Deficient knowledge

Nursing Diagnosis	Rationale	Nursing Interventions

Three hours later, Mrs. FJM's family comes to the nursing station to say that Mrs. FJM is having difficulty breathing. You go into Mrs. FJM's room and assess the following: complaints of chest pain, R 36, P 134, BP 108/88, pulse ox 90%, coughing, dyspnea, anxiousness.

On the basis of the situation **3 hours later,** identify and write the **priority problem** in the box below. Then, starting with the small box labeled **#1, prioritize** the **nursing interventions** for this situation and **identify** your follow-up action plan for Mrs. FJM.

NURSING INTERVENTIONS   **DECISION-MAKING DIAGRAM**

A. Stay with Mrs. FJM

B. Raise head of bed

C. Take P, R, BP, assess pain level

D. Monitor oxygen saturation level

E. Notify MD

F. Administer oxygen

New Action Plan

#1 #2 #3 #4 #5 #6

Priority Problem

NOTES

2-7 THE PATIENT WITH CIRRHOSIS OF THE LIVER

1600 Handoff Report:

| **S** | You are assigned to care for Mr. U, 46 years old, admitted with the diagnosis of Laënnec cirrhosis. He is jaundiced, has ascites, and has increasing shortness of breath. His VS at 12:00 PM were T 99°F, P 94, R 34, BP 140/90, pulse ox 96%, pain level 0. The vital signs are consistent with previous recordings. |

It is now 1630 and the following patient care plan information is available:

VS q4h I & O (✓) Neuro cks q4h CBC, serum ammonia ⎰ AST, ALT, PT ⎱ today Procedure: Abd paracentesis at 5:00 PM today	Saline lock (✓) Bed rest with BRP Weigh daily Measure abd girth daily Code status: Full	Diet: ↑ CHO, 30 g prot., 2 g Na⁺ Routine med: Aluminum hydroxide 30 mL po 10-2-6-10 Furosemide 40 mg IVP qAM Spironolactone 50 mg po bid

Prioritize the five **recommended nursing interventions** as you would do them to take care of Mr. U. Write a number in the box to identify the order of your interventions (#1 = first intervention, #2 = second intervention, etc.), and state a **rationale** for each intervention.

INTERVENTIONS	PRIORITY #	RATIONALE
• Ensure that consent form is signed	☐	_____
• Take the vital signs	☐	_____
• Perform a body systems physical	☐	_____
• Ensure that abdominal paracentesis equipment is on the unit	☐	_____
• Have Mr. U void	☐	_____

KEY POINTS TO CONSIDER _____

_____

_____

The physician performs the abdominal paracentesis on Mr. U and removes 2.5 L of fluid. VS during the procedure were P 90, R 32, BP 136/86. Postprocedure you assess:
1. VS: P 94, R 24, BP 136/86, pain level 1
2. Dressing at the abdominal puncture site is clean
3. Mr. U is lying in a semi-Fowler position
4. He is alert and oriented, although slow to respond

Collaborative Learning Activity: With a partner, **do the following: (1) select the one nursing diagnosis** that is a priority at this time, **(2) provide a rationale** for your selection, and **(3) list the nursing interventions** that assist you to meet the needs of the patient.

All of the following nursing diagnoses may apply to Mr. U:

Risk for falls, Risk for infection, Impaired skin integrity, Impaired physical mobility, Acute pain, Imbalanced nutrition: less than body requirements, Risk for activity intolerance, Impaired tissue integrity, Excess fluid volume, Risk for deficient fluid volume, Ineffective breathing pattern, Disturbed body image, Disturbed sleep pattern, Fatigue, Impaired comfort

Nursing Diagnosis	Rationale	Nursing Interventions

The **laboratory results** for today are:

PT 40 sec	Serum ammonia 70 µg/dL	Hgb 10.6 g/dL	Hct 30%
WBC 3500/mm^3	Platelets 100,000/mm^3	AST 100 U/L	ALT 500 U/L

Based on the **laboratory results**, identify and write the **priority problem** in the box below. Then, starting with the small box labeled **#1, prioritize** the **nursing interventions** for this situation and **identify** your follow-up action plan for Mr. U.

NURSING INTERVENTIONS

A. Monitor the VS

B. Assess for petechiae

C. Check stool for occult blood

D. Monitor urine color

E. Check neuro status

F. Notify MD

DECISION-MAKING DIAGRAM

New Action Plan

#1 #2 #3 #4 #5 #6

☐ ☐ ☐ ☐ ☐ ☐

Priority Problem

NOTES _____

APPLYING CRITICAL THINKING SKILLS TO TEST QUESTIONS

INSTRUCTIONS: Circle the one best answer for each test question. Write your rationale for selecting the answer. To enhance your learning and test-taking skills, discuss your answer and rationale with a partner. The answer and the rationale can be found on the back of this page.

2 Priority Setting and Decision Making

1. The physician orders phytonadione (vitamin K) 10 mg IM for an adult client with liver cirrhosis and ascites. Available is a vial of phytonadione 10 mg/mL. The nurse is planning to administer this dose in the deltoid. Which of the following is most appropriate for the administration of the ordered amount to the client?
   a. 1-mL syringe with 25-gauge 5/8-inch needle
   b. 1-mL syringe with 23-gauge 1/2-inch needle
   c. 3-mL syringe with 23-gauge 1-inch needle
   d. 3-mL syringe with 22-gauge 1 1/2-inch needle

   Rationale for your selection: _____
   _____
   _____
   _____

2. The nurse admits a client with cirrhosis of the liver and severe ascites. The client is oriented, jaundiced, and complains of itching. Respirations are 28, short, and shallow. Urine is dark amber. Which action is most important for the nurse to consider?
   a. Sit client in high Fowler's position.
   b. Encourage client to drink more fluids.
   c. Limit client activity.
   d. Assess skin integrity daily.

   Rationale for your selection: _____
   _____
   _____
   _____

3. The client is admitted with cirrhosis of the liver and ascites. The physician orders the administration of an IV infusion of albumin. Which of the following is the expected outcome after the administration of the albumin?
   a. Decreased complaints of pruritus
   b. Decreased serum ammonia levels
   c. Increased secretion of sodium
   d. Increased urinary output

   Rationale for your selection: _____
   _____
   _____
   _____

ANSWER KEY FOR
APPLYING CRITICAL THINKING SKILLS TO TEST QUESTIONS

HELPFUL HINTS: Read all test questions carefully. Identify key words in the question that will guide you in answering the question. In these test questions the **key words** to consider are **"most appropriate," "most important,"** and **"expected outcome."** Compare your rationale with the one in the test question.

1. The physician orders phytonadione (vitamin K) 10 mg IM for an adult client with liver cirrhosis and ascites. Available is a vial of phytonadione 10 mg/mL. The nurse is planning to administer this dose in the deltoid. Which of the following is most appropriate for the administration of the ordered amount to the client?
   a. 1-mL syringe with 25-gauge 5/8-inch needle
   b. 1-mL syringe with 23-gauge 1/2-inch needle
   c. 3-mL syringe with 23-gauge 1-inch needle
   d. 3-mL syringe with 22-gauge 1 1/2-inch needle

Rationale: The answer is (c). It is most appropriate to use a smaller IM needle gauge because clients with liver cirrhosis are at a high risk for bleeding. The deltoid is a smaller muscle than the gluteus, so a 1-inch needle is the best choice. Options (a), (b), and (d) are not the best choice for this client.

2. The nurse admits a client with cirrhosis of the liver and severe ascites. The client is oriented, jaundiced, and complains of itching. Respirations are 28, short, and shallow. Urine is dark amber. Which action is most important for the nurse to consider?
   a. Sit client in high Fowler's position.
   b. Encourage client to drink more fluids.
   c. Limit client activity.
   d. Assess skin integrity daily.

Rationale: The answer is (c). Activity increases the metabolic needs of the body, thereby increasing the workload of the liver. Option (a) is not the most appropriate position for a client with severe ascites because it compromises respiration. Options (b) and (d) are not the most important interventions.

3. The client is admitted with cirrhosis of the liver and ascites. The physician orders the administration of an IV infusion of albumin. Which of the following is the expected outcome after the administration of the albumin?
   a. Decreased complaints of pruritus
   b. Decreased serum ammonia levels
   c. Increased secretion of sodium
   d. Increased urinary output

Rationale: The answer is (d). Albumin increases plasma colloid osmotic pressure, thereby increasing diuresis. Options (a), (b), and (c) are not expected outcomes for this ordered intervention.

2-8 THE PATIENT WITH HEPATIC ENCEPHALOPATHY

0700 Handoff Report:

S	Mr. U, 47 years old, is admitted with the diagnosis of hepatic encephalopathy related to his advanced cirrhosis of the liver. This is his second admission. He was awake most of the night, very restless, and confused to time and place. VS at 0400 were T 97°F Ax, P 88, R 22, BP 120/88, pulse ox 92%. Unable to assess pain level but every effort has been made to keep him comfortable. ⚠️ A patient care assistant was in his room most of the shift. Mr. U is less restless this morning.

The following patient care plan information is available:

VS q4h I & O (✓) Neuro cks q4h Serum ammonia, K⁺ today Code status: No code	D5W @ 100 mL/hr #20 g RFA—inserted today Bed rest with BRP Weigh daily	Diet: ↑ CHO, 50 g Prot., 2 g Na⁺ Routine med: Neomycin 1 g po q6h Lactulose 30 mL po bid

Prioritize the following five **recommended nursing interventions** as you would do them to take care of Mr. U. Write a number in the box to identify the order of your interventions (#1 = first intervention, #2 = second intervention, etc.), and state a **rationale** for each intervention.

INTERVENTIONS	PRIORITY #	Rationale
• Take VS	☐	_____ _____ _____
• Assess level of consciousness and orientation	☐	_____ _____ _____
• Check current serum ammonia and K⁺ levels	☐	_____ _____ _____
• Perform a body systems physical assessment	☐	_____ _____ _____
• Assist Mr. U with his activities of daily living and provide comfort care	☐	_____ _____ _____

KEY POINTS TO CONSIDER _____

_____

_____

_____

2 Priority Setting and Decision Making

Mr. U has refused his morning dose of lactulose and you further assess:
1. He refused the lactulose the previous day
2. No bowel movement for 2 days
3. Irritable, speech slurred
4. Responds slowly to verbal communication

Collaborative Learning Activity: With a partner, **do the following: (1) select the one nursing diagnosis** that is a priority at this time, **(2) provide a rationale** for your selection, and **(3) list the nursing interventions** that assist you to meet the needs of the patient.

All of the following nursing diagnoses may apply to Mr. U:

Risk for falls, Risk for infection, Impaired skin integrity, Bathing self-care deficit, Impaired physical mobility, Constipation, Imbalanced nutrition: less than body requirements, Activity intolerance, Impaired tissue integrity, Excess fluid volume, Ineffective breathing pattern, Fatigue, Disturbed sleep pattern, Impaired comfort

Nursing Diagnosis	Rationale	Nursing Interventions

You return from lunch at 1 PM and are informed of the following: Mr. U is becoming increasingly confused and lethargic. He did not eat lunch.

Based on the 1 PM information, identify and write the **priority problem** in the box below. Then, starting with the small box labeled **#1, prioritize** the **nursing interventions** for this situation and **identify** your follow-up action plan for Mr. U.

NURSING INTERVENTIONS

A. Inform physician

B. Record assessment findings

C. Take VS, pulse ox

D. Monitor neurologic status

E. Stay with patient

F. Raise the bedrails

DECISION-MAKING DIAGRAM

New Action Plan

#1 #2 #3 #4 #5 #6

Priority Problem

NOTES _____

_____

APPLYING CRITICAL THINKING SKILLS TO TEST QUESTIONS

INSTRUCTIONS: Circle the one best answer for each test question. Write your rationale for selecting the answer. To enhance your learning and test-taking skills, discuss your answer and rationale with a partner. The answer and the rationale can be found on the back of this page.

1. The client is diagnosed with hepatic encephalopathy and is receiving lactulose 30 mL po bid. To effectively monitor the therapeutic effects of the drug therapy, the nurse would primarily assess for a(n)
   a. decrease in abdominal girth.
   b. increase in bowel movements.
   c. increase in serum albumin levels.
   d. decrease in serum ammonia levels.

   Rationale for your selection: _____
   _____
   _____
   _____

2. The nurse administers spironolactone 100 mg po to a client with portal hypertension. Which of the following is most important for the nurse to monitor during the administration of this drug?
   a. Serum potassium levels
   b. Intake and output
   c. Specific gravity of urine
   d. Abdominal girth

   Rationale for your selection: _____
   _____
   _____
   _____

3. The nurse is caring for a client admitted with portal hypertension and ascites. Which assessment finding is most indicative of a serious complication?
   a. Caput medusae noted on abdomen
   b. Complaints of fatigue and weakness
   c. Hematemesis after breakfast
   d. 2-lb weight loss from previous day

   Rationale for your selection: _____
   _____
   _____
   _____

ANSWER KEY FOR
APPLYING CRITICAL THINKING SKILLS TO TEST QUESTIONS

HELPFUL HINTS: Read all test questions carefully. Identify key words in the question that will guide you in answering the question. In these test questions the **key words** to consider are **"primarily," "most important,"** and **"most indicative."** Compare your rationale with the one in the test question.

1. The client is diagnosed with hepatic encephalopathy and is receiving lactulose 30 mL po bid. To effectively monitor the therapeutic effects of the drug therapy, the nurse would primarily assess for a(n)
   a. decrease in abdominal girth.
   b. increase in bowel movements.
   c. increase in serum albumin levels.
   d. decrease in serum ammonia levels.

Rationale: The answer is (d). The expected therapeutic effect for this client is to decrease serum ammonia levels by trapping ammonium ions in the intestine and excreting them in the stool. Options (a) and (c) do not provide the nurse with the therapeutic drug effects, and option (b) is not as specific a measure of effectiveness as the serum ammonia level.

2. The nurse administers spironolactone 100 mg po to a client with portal hypertension. Which of the following is most important for the nurse to monitor during the administration of this drug?
   a. Serum potassium levels
   b. Intake and output
   c. Specific gravity of urine
   d. Abdominal girth

Rationale: The answer is (a). Serum potassium levels should be monitored when a client is on spironolactone, a potassium-sparing diuretic. Options (b), (c), and (d) are not the most important interventions.

3. The nurse is caring for a client admitted with portal hypertension and ascites. Which assessment finding is most indicative of a serious complication?
   a. Caput medusae noted on abdomen
   b. Complaints of fatigue and weakness
   c. Hematemesis after breakfast
   d. 2-lb weight loss from previous day

Rationale: The answer is (c). Clients with portal hypertension may also have esophageal varices. The client should be monitored for further signs of bleeding. Option (a) is an expected finding consistent with ascites. Option (b) needs further assessment, and option (d) is not most indicative of a serious complication.

2-9 THE PATIENT WITH DIABETES MELLITUS

0700 Handoff Report:

S	Mrs. G, a 56-year-old Hispanic female, was admitted with the diagnosis of end-stage renal disease (ESRD). She takes isophane NPH insulin 25 units subcut qAM and isophane NPH insulin 15 units in the evening. The blood glucose fingersticks are ordered a.c. and 2100. She is scheduled to have hemodialysis this AM. Breakfast arrives at 0800.
B	Mrs. G has a 30-year history of diabetes mellitus type 1. She has experienced neuropathy and visual changes.
A	Vital signs this morning are: T 36°C, P 80, R 18, BP 154/92, pulse ox 94%, pain level 0. BG was done and recorded. Mrs. G has a 2-cm dry, ulcerated circular area on the lateral outer aspect of her right great toe and an arteriovenous (AV) fistula in the right forearm. The AV fistula is patent with a strong thrill and bruit.
R	The following nursing interventions are recommended:

Prioritize the following five **recommended nursing interventions** as you would do them to initially take care of Mrs. G. Write a number in the box to identify the order of your interventions (#1 = first intervention, #2 = second intervention, etc.), and state a **rationale** for each intervention.

INTERVENTIONS	PRIORITY #	RATIONALE
• Check for the fingerstick blood glucose	☐	_____
• Assess AV fistula	☐	_____
• Administer isophane NPH insulin 25 units subcut	☐	_____
• Give patient breakfast	☐	_____
• Perform a body systems physical assessment	☐	_____

KEY POINTS TO CONSIDER _____

_____

_____

2 Priority Setting and Decision Making

Mrs. G is still waiting for her dialysis treatment. Correction insulin scale (sliding scale) for finger-stick blood glucose:	At 1000 the physician leaves the following orders: 251–275 give 6 units insulin lispro. 211–250 give 4 units insulin lispro. 150–210 give 2 units insulin lispro. Less than 150 no insulin.

You do a BG fingerstick at 1145. The BG results are 215. You will give _____ insulin lispro within 15 minutes before lunch.

⚙ **Collaborative Learning Activity:** With a partner, **do the following: (1) select the one nursing diagnosis** that is a priority at this time, **(2) provide a rationale** for your selection, and **(3) list the nursing interventions** that assist you to meet the needs of the patient.

All of the following nursing diagnoses may apply to Mrs. G:

Risk for infection, Risk for impaired skin integrity, Impaired physical mobility, Ineffective sexuality patterns, Fatigue, Excess fluid volume, Deficient fluid volume, Imbalanced nutrition: less than body requirements

Nursing Diagnosis	Rationale	Nursing Interventions

As you take her 1300 VS, you assess the following signs and symptoms: irritability, skin warm, moist, VS: T 36.8°C, P 100, R 18, BP 150/84. She complains of dizziness and "feeling funny." You suspect a hypoglycemic reaction.

On the basis of the situation above, identify and write the **priority problem** in the box below. Then, starting with the small box labeled **#1, prioritize** the **nursing interventions** for this situation and **identify** your plan for follow-up care for Mrs. G.

NURSING INTERVENTIONS   **DECISION-MAKING DIAGRAM**

A. Record findings/nursing care

B. Do a fingerstick blood glucose stat

C. Check fingerstick blood glucose in 15 minutes

New Action Plan
#1 #2 #3 #4 #5 #6

D. Prepare to give 4 ounces of apple juice

E. Alert the RN stat

F. Raise the side rails

Priority Problem

NOTES _____

APPLYING CRITICAL THINKING SKILLS TO TEST QUESTIONS

INSTRUCTIONS: Circle the one best answer for each test question. Write your rationale for selecting the answer. To enhance your learning and test-taking skills, discuss your answer and rationale with a partner. The answer and the rationale can be found on the back of this page.

1. The nurse is providing discharge instructions to a newly diagnosed client with type 1 diabetes mellitus who will take 5 units regular insulin and 10 units isophane NPH insulin qAM. The client informs the nurse that he runs 2 miles every morning. In teaching the client about insulin absorption and exercise, it is important for the nurse to teach the client to
   a. inject the morning dose of insulin into the abdomen.
   b. hold the morning dose of regular insulin until after the exercise.
   c. hold the morning dose of isophane NPH insulin until after the exercise.
   d. inject the morning dose of insulin into the lower extremity.

   Rationale for your selection: _____
   _____
   _____
   _____

2. The nurse notes the following medications on a client's medication record: Isophane NPH insulin 13 units subcut qAM at 0730 and lispro 5 units subcut at the start of breakfast. The breakfast arrives at 0830 on the unit. In assessing the medication record, which action by the nurse is most appropriate?
   a. Question the lispro insulin order.
   b. Question the isophane NPH insulin order.
   c. Give both insulins at 0730 in one syringe.
   d. Give the insulins as ordered.

   Rationale for your selection: _____
   _____
   _____
   _____

3. The nurse is preparing to draw up insulin glargine 12 units using a low-dose insulin syringe. Which technique indicates the most appropriate procedure before giving the insulin? The nurse takes the medication record and the insulin syringe with the 12 units of insulin and
   a. checks the drawn-up dose with another nurse.
   b. with the syringe in the vial, checks the drawn-up dose with another nurse.
   c. takes the vial of insulin to check the drawn-up dose with another nurse.
   d. double-checks by charting the dose of insulin before injecting the insulin.

   Rationale for your selection: _____
   _____
   _____
   _____

ANSWER KEY FOR
APPLYING CRITICAL THINKING SKILLS TO TEST QUESTIONS

HELPFUL HINTS: Read all test questions carefully. Identify key words in the question that will guide you in answering the question. In these test questions the **key words** to consider are **"absorption and exercise"** and **"most appropriate."** Compare your rationale with the one in the test question.

1. The nurse is providing discharge instructions to a newly diagnosed client with type 1 diabetes mellitus who will take 5 units regular insulin and 10 units isophane NPH insulin qAM. The client informs the nurse that he runs 2 miles every morning. In teaching the client about insulin absorption and exercise, it is important for the nurse to teach the client to
   a. inject the morning dose of insulin into the abdomen.
   b. hold the morning dose of regular human insulin until after the exercise.
   c. hold the morning dose of isophane NPH insulin until after the exercise.
   d. inject the morning dose of insulin into the lower extremity.

Rationale: The answer is (a). The abdomen is a better injection site because the absorption rate of insulin is faster when injected into an extremity that is exercised. Options (b), (c), and (d) do not correlate the effects of diabetes, insulin therapy, and exercise.

2. The nurse notes the following medications on a client's medication record: Isophane NPH insulin 13 units subcut qAM at 0730 and lispro 5 units subcut at the start of breakfast. The breakfast arrives at 0830 on the unit. In assessing the medication record, which action by the nurse is most appropriate?
   a. Question the lispro insulin order.
   b. Question the isophane NPH insulin order.
   c. Give both insulins at 0730 in one syringe.
   d. Give the insulins as ordered.

Rationale: The answer is (d). It is most appropriate to consider that lispro is a rapid-acting insulin with an onset of 10 to 15 minutes and should be administered at the start of the meal. Options (a), (b), and (c) do not address the onset of action of the rapid-acting insulin.

3. The nurse is preparing to draw up insulin glargine 12 units using a low-dose insulin syringe. Which technique indicates the most appropriate procedure before giving the insulin? The nurse takes the medication record and the insulin syringe with the 12 units of insulin and
   a. checks the drawn-up dose with another nurse.
   b. with the syringe in the vial, checks the drawn-up dose with another nurse.
   c. takes the vial of insulin to check the drawn-up dose with another nurse.
   d. double-checks by charting the dose of insulin before injecting the insulin.

Rationale: The answer is (b). To prevent a medication error, it is recommended that the syringe remain in the insulin vial when checking the type and dose of insulin with another nurse. Options (a), (c), and (d) are not the most appropriate and recommended procedure.

2-10 THE PATIENT UNDERGOING HEMODIALYSIS

0700 Handoff Report:

S	Ms. A, 52 years old, has ESRD and has just been started on dialysis. She has an AV fistula in the right forearm and is scheduled for hemodialysis at 0800 today. Patient has not been weighed this morning. The AV fistula has a strong thrill and bruit. Ms. A's BP is 160/102.

The following patient care plan information is available:

VS q8h I & O (✓) Hemodialysis today Weigh daily Hgb & Hct (✓) Serum ferritin (✓) Serum iron saturation (✓) Electrolytes (Na⁺, K⁺, CL⁻, CO₂)	IV: Saline lock—left hand Routine medications: Enalapril 10 mg po qAM 0800 Folic acid 1 mg po qAM 0800 FeSO₄ 325 po tid c̄ meals Epoetin alfa 30,000 units subcut M-W-F	Diet: 70 g protein, 2 g Na⁺, 2 g K⁺ Fluid restriction 1000 mL/day

Prioritize the following five **recommended nursing interventions** as you would do them to take care of Ms. A. Write a number in the box to identify the order of your interventions (#1 = first intervention, #2 = second intervention, etc.), and state a **rationale** for each intervention.

INTERVENTIONS	PRIORITY #	RATIONALE
⚠ • Take the VS (BP on the left arm)	☐	_____
• Perform body systems physical assessment	☐	_____
• Weigh patient	☐	_____
• Assess AV fistula for thrill and bruit	☐	_____
• Hold folic acid and enalapril	☐	_____

KEY POINTS TO CONSIDER _____

_____

_____

Ordered laboratory studies were drawn before dialysis. The results of the morning laboratory tests are:
1. Hemoglobin 9.5 g/dL, hematocrit 28%
2. Ferritin 60 ng/mL
3. Serum iron saturation 18%
4. K^+ 5.0 mEq

Collaborative Learning Activity: With a partner, **do the following: (1) select the one nursing diagnosis** that is a priority at this time, **(2) provide a rationale** for your selection, and **(3) list the nursing interventions** that assist you to meet the needs of the patient.

All of the following nursing diagnoses may apply to Ms. A:

Risk for injury, Deficient knowledge, Fear, Anxiety, Risk for infection, Impaired tissue integrity, Constipation, Excess fluid volume, Deficient fluid volume, Disturbed body image, Impaired physical mobility, Ineffective peripheral tissue perfusion, Imbalanced nutrition: less than body requirements, Fatigue

Nursing Diagnosis	Rationale	Nursing Interventions

After the dialysis treatment, Ms. A is restless and you assess: Complains of headache, pruritus, nausea, change in level of consciousness, muscle twitching, confusion.

On the basis of data **after the dialysis treatment,** identify and write the **priority problem** in the box below. Then, starting with the small box labeled **#1, prioritize** the **nursing interventions** for this situation and **identify** your follow-up action plan for Ms. A.

NURSING INTERVENTIONS

A. Take the VS

B. Notify physician

C. Maintain calm, quiet environment

D. Stay with patient

E. Monitor neurologic status

F. Record assessment findings

DECISION-MAKING DIAGRAM

New Action Plan

#1   #2   #3   #4   #5   #6

☐   ☐   ☐   ☐   ☐   ☐

Priority Problem

NOTES _____

APPLYING CRITICAL THINKING SKILLS TO TEST QUESTIONS

INSTRUCTIONS: Circle the one best answer for each test question. Write your rationale for selecting the answer. To enhance your learning and test-taking skills, discuss your answer and rationale with a partner. The answer and the rationale can be found on the back of this page.

1. Which statement made by a newly diagnosed patient with chronic kidney disease requires further explanation?
   a. "I understand that my chronic kidney disease may progress to end-stage renal disease."
   b. "By controlling my hypertension, I can help control the damage to the kidneys."
   c. "It may be years before my chronic kidney disease become worse."
   d. "I understand that the damage to my kidneys can be reversed."

   Rationale for your selection: _____
   _____
   _____
   _____

2. The nurse administers epoetin alfa 10,000 units subcut twice weekly to the client with ESRD. The most effective method of evaluating the therapeutic effect of epoetin alfa is for the nurse to assess for
   a. a decrease in skin pallor.
   b. an increase in client activity.
   c. an increase in the hematocrit level.
   d. a decrease in complaints of weakness and fatigue.

   Rationale for your selection: _____
   _____
   _____
   _____

3. The nurse is caring for a client scheduled for hemodialysis this morning. In preparing the client for the dialysis treatment, it is most important for the nurse to
   a. allow the client to rest until after the dialysis treatment.
   b. ensure that all morning care is completed before dialysis.
   c. make the client NPO until after the dialysis treatment.
   d. withhold the morning dose of any antihypertensive drugs.

   Rationale for your selection: _____
   _____
   _____
   _____

ANSWER KEY FOR
APPLYING CRITICAL THINKING SKILLS TO TEST QUESTIONS

HELPFUL HINTS: Read all test questions carefully. Identify key words in the question that will guide you in answering the question. In these test questions the **key words** to consider are **"priority," "most effective,"** and **"most important."** Compare your rationale with the one in the test question.

1. Which statement made by a newly diagnosed patient with chronic kidney disease requires further explanation?
   a. "I understand that my chronic kidney disease may progress to end-stage renal disease."
   b. "By controlling my hypertension, I can help control the damage to the kidneys."
   c. "It may be years before my chronic kidney disease become worse."
   d. "I understand that the damage to my kidneys can be reversed."

Rationale: The answer is (d). Kidney damage cannot be reversed but it can be controlled. Options (a), (b), and (c) are correct statements related to the progression and control of chronic kidney (renal) failure.

2. The nurse administers epoetin alfa 10,000 units subcut twice weekly to the client with ESRD. The most effective method of evaluating the therapeutic effect of epoetin alfa is for the nurse to assess for
   a. a decrease in skin pallor.
   b. an increase in client activity.
   c. an increase in the hematocrit level.
   d. a decrease in complaints of weakness and fatigue.

Rationale: The answer is (c). Epoetin alfa stimulates the production of red blood cells. The hematocrit is an indirect measurement of the total number and volume of red blood cells. Options (a), (b), and (d) may be manifested as a result of the rise in the number of red blood cells.

3. The nurse is caring for a client scheduled for hemodialysis this morning. In preparing the client for the dialysis treatment, it is most important for the nurse to
   a. allow the client to rest until after the dialysis treatment.
   b. ensure that all morning care is completed before dialysis.
   c. make the client NPO until after the dialysis treatment.
   d. withhold the morning dose of any antihypertensive drugs.

Rationale: The answer is (d). Hypotension is a complication of dialysis. Antihypertensive drugs taken before dialysis can cause severe hypotension. Options (a) and (b) are not the most important in preparing the client, and option (c) is not necessary in preparing the client for hemodialysis.

2-11 THE PATIENT WITH PERIPHERAL ARTERIAL DISEASE

1500 Handoff Report:

S	Mr. L, 70 years old, is sent to the hospital after visiting his physician with complaints of increasing painful muscle cramps after ambulating. He needs to be admitted, and the following orders are available.

VS q4h I & O (✓) Pedal pulse check q4h Bed rest with BRP CBC, UA, Electrolytes Mr. L Age: 70	Insert saline lock Drsg chgs: Clean ulcerated area on left lateral ankle with NS—apply dry sterile 4 × 4s (Wound care specialist to assess today ⚙) Dx: Peripheral artery disease	Diet: mech soft Routine med: Pentoxifylline 400 mg po tid Aspirin 81 mg po daily

On assessing Mr. L, you note that he is alert but hard of hearing. He has a bandage around his left foot. He tells you he uses this to keep his shoe from rubbing his foot. He has another bandage over his left ankle. He lives alone, and his medical history is significant for hypertension.

Prioritize the following five **recommended nursing interventions** as you would do them to take care of Mr. L. Write a number in the box to identify the order of your interventions (#1 = first intervention, #2 = second intervention, etc.), and state a **rationale** for each intervention.

INTERVENTIONS	PRIORITY #	RATIONALE
• Take the VS, pulse ox, assess pain level	☐	_____
• Assess bilateral pedal pulses	☐	_____
• Orient to hospital room	☐	_____
• Perform a body systems assessment	☐	_____
• Apply sterile dressing to left ankle	☐	_____

KEY POINTS TO CONSIDER _____

_____

_____

You assist Mr. L to the bathroom; on his return to bed you note the following:
1. Bilateral lower extremities—reddish blue in color
2. Bilateral pedal pulses weak (1+), capillary refill greater than 3 seconds
3. The skin of the lower extremities is cool, tight, and shiny
4. Gait slow, needs assistance

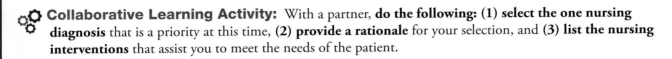 **Collaborative Learning Activity:** With a partner, **do the following: (1) select the one nursing diagnosis** that is a priority at this time, **(2) provide a rationale** for your selection, and **(3) list the nursing interventions** that assist you to meet the needs of the patient.

All of the following nursing diagnoses may apply to Mr. L:

Risk for injury: fall, Deficient knowledge, Risk for infection, Impaired skin integrity, Impaired physical mobility, Ineffective peripheral tissue perfusion, Activity intolerance, Impaired tissue integrity, Acute pain

Nursing Diagnosis	Rationale	Nursing Interventions

After having changed the dressing on the left ankle, you **remove the bandage** from the left foot and you note: two discolored shrunken black toes.

Based on the observation noted after the **removal of the bandages,** identify and write the **priority problem** in the box below. Then, starting with the small box labeled **#1, prioritize** the **nursing interventions** for this situation and **identify** your follow-up action plan for Mr. L.

NURSING INTERVENTIONS

DECISION-MAKING DIAGRAM

A. Assess pain level

B. Measure blackened area

C. Put on sterile gloves

D. Cleanse area with normal saline

E. Apply sterile dressing

F. Record assessment findings

New Action Plan

#1 #2 #3 #4 #5 #6

Priority Problem

NOTES

2-12 THE PATIENT WITH CHEST PAIN

0700 Handoff Report:

S	Mrs. T, 56 years old, was admitted around midnight from the ER after experiencing some chest pain. Mrs. T has been taking verapamil, nifedipine, and atenolol. Mrs. T will continue with her usual cardiac and blood pressure medications and is also started on aspirin 81 mg, docusate sodium, lovastatin, and aluminum hydroxide 15 mL after meals and at the hour of sleep. PRN medications include nitroglycerin tablets 0.4 mg SL every 5 minutes for up to 3 doses prn chest pain, and morphine sulfate 4 mg IV push if chest pain not relieved with the nitroglycerin. She has bathroom privileges with assistance, a saline lock, and oxygen at 3 L/min/nasal cannula to keep the oxygen saturation greater than 96%. Mrs. T is upset about not being able to get up and smoke.
B	She has coronary artery disease and smokes one pack of cigarettes a day. Her father died of heart disease and she has a brother with hypertension.
A	Her VS are T 98°F, P 90, R 26, BP 164/100, pain level 0, pulse ox 97%. Mrs. T is requesting to use the commode as you start your shift.
R	The following nursing interventions are recommended:

Prioritize the following five **recommended nursing interventions** as you would do them to initially take care of Mrs. T. Write a number in the box to identify the order of your interventions (#1 = first intervention, #2 = second intervention, etc.), and state a **rationale** for each intervention.

INTERVENTIONS	PRIORITY #	RATIONALE
• Take the vital signs and assess pain level	☐	_____
• Assist to commode	☐	_____
• Perform a body systems assessment	☐	_____
• Check oxygen saturation level	☐	_____
• Talk with Mrs. T	☐	_____

KEY POINTS TO CONSIDER _____

_____

_____

After breakfast Mrs. T continues to be upset. She states that she is constipated and above all wants to smoke. She is getting increasingly upset. You observe the following:

1. Abdomen round, bowel sounds present in all four quadrants
2. Breakfast intake 30%
3. Last bowel movement 2 days ago
4. SOB, oxygen saturation at 93%

⚙ **Collaborative Learning Activity:** With a partner, **do the following: (1) select the one nursing diagnosis** that is a priority at this time, **(2) provide a rationale** for your selection, and **(3) list the nursing interventions** that assist you to meet the needs of the patient.

All of the following nursing diagnoses may apply to Mrs. T:

Acute pain, Deficient knowledge, Anxiety, Noncompliance, Ineffective coping, Decreased cardiac output, Activity intolerance, Risk for impaired skin integrity, Constipation, Ineffective health maintenance

Nursing Diagnosis	Rationale	Nursing Interventions

At **10:00 AM** the nursing assistant reports that Mrs. T is feeling chest pain. You assess and note that she has cool, clammy skin and complains of indigestion and tightness in her chest. BP 154/98, P 100, R 30, states chest pain at a level of 8. Oxygen saturation is 88%.

On the basis of the data at **10:00 AM,** identify and write the **priority problem** in the box below. Then, starting with the small box labeled **#1, prioritize** the **nursing interventions** for this situation and **identify** your follow-up action plan for Mrs. T.

NURSING INTERVENTIONS

A. Oxygen @ 3 L/min/NC

⚙ B. Activate the hospital's Rapid Response Team

C. Administer nitroglycerin 0.4 mg SL tab i q5min ×3

D. Monitor VS q5min

E. Obtain 12-lead electrocardiogram per protocol

F. Notify physician

DECISION-MAKING DIAGRAM

New Action Plan

#1 #2 #3 #4 #5 #6

Priority Problem

NOTES _____

2-13 THE PATIENT WITH HEART FAILURE

1000 Transfer Handoff Report:

> **S** Mr. T is transferred to the telemetry unit from the emergency room. He is diagnosed with heart failure (HF). He has 3+ pitting edema of the lower extremities and increasing shortness of breath. He has been demonstrating Cheyne-Stokes respirations periods of confusion and complains of blurred vision.
> Vital signs are T 97.6°F, P 62, R 22, BP 180/102, pain level 0, pulse ox 96%. He has received his 0900 meds.

The following patient care plan information is available:

VS q4h I & O (✓) Up in chair qid O$_2$ @ 3 L/min/NP Serum K$^+$, PT, PTT, ABG (✓) Chest x-ray (✓) ECG (✓) Name: T. Age: 72	IV D5W @ 50 mL/hr IV site: LFA #20 g LBM: 2 days ago Foley (✓) Code status: Full code Dx: Heart failure	Diet: Soft (NAS) Routine medications: Digoxin 0.25 mg IVP qAM 0900 Furosemide 40 mg po bid 0900–1700 Docusate sodium 100 mg tab i po qAM 0900 Prazosin HCl 10 mg po bid 0900–1700

Prioritize the following five **recommended interventions** as you would do them to take care of Mr. T. Write a number in the box to identify the order of your interventions (#1 = first intervention, #2 = second intervention, etc.), and state a **rationale** for each intervention.

INTERVENTIONS	PRIORITY #	RATIONALE
• Assess respiratory rate	☐	
• Obtain urinary output data	☐	
• Assess rate/rhythm and quality	☐	
• Assess visual complaints	☐	
• Check current lab data	☐	

KEY POINTS TO CONSIDER _____

Mr. T wants to wash up, but he says that he does not have the energy like he used to and that he gets tired very easily. You assist him with morning care and assess the following:

1. Skin cool, dusky in color
2. Lower extremities with 2+ pitting edema
3. Lung sounds with crackles on inspiration; R 24, regular pattern
4. Alert and oriented at this time

Collaborative Learning Activity: With a partner, **do the following: (1) select the one nursing diagnosis** that is a priority at this time, **(2) provide a rationale** for your selection, and **(3) list the nursing interventions** that assist you to meet the needs of the patient.

All of the following nursing diagnoses may apply to Mr. T:

> Anxiety, Risk for infection, Activity intolerance, Excess fluid volume, Impaired tissue integrity, Risk for ineffective cerebral tissue perfusion, Imbalanced nutrition: less than body requirements, Risk for injury, Deficient knowledge, Impaired gas exchange, Fatigue

Nursing Diagnosis	Rationale	Nursing Interventions

Mr. T's family stops to visit during lunch. **At 1:00 PM,** the nursing assistant tells you that Mr. T is in distress. You walk into the room and notice Mr. T holding his chest tightly. Shortly afterward you assess: cyanosis, no pulse, no BP, and no respirations.

On the basis of the situation at **1:00 PM,** identify and write the **priority problem** in the box below. Then, starting with the small box labeled **#1, prioritize** the **nursing interventions** for this situation and **identify** your follow-up action plan for Mr. T.

NURSING INTERVENTIONS

A. Call the Code Team/Rapid Response Team

B. Place in supine position

C. Begin CPR

D. Notify physician

E. Record findings

F. Support family

DECISION-MAKING DIAGRAM

New Action Plan

#1 #2 #3 #4 #5 #6

Priority Problem

NOTES _____

_____

APPLYING CRITICAL THINKING SKILLS TO TEST QUESTIONS

INSTRUCTIONS: Circle the one best answer for each test question. Write your rationale for selecting the answer. To enhance your learning and test-taking skills, discuss your answer and rationale with a partner. The answer and the rationale can be found on the back of this page.

1. The nurse admits a 69-year-old male client with heart failure. The physician orders furosemide 60 mg IVP stat, digoxin 0.25 mg po, and KCl 20 mEq po now. Which assessment finding is most indicative of an ineffective response 2 hours after the administration of all the medications?
   a. Pulse 89, irregular
   b. Urine output 60 mL
   c. Pulse oximetry 94%
   d. Pitting edema in the lower extremities

   Rationale for your selection: _____
   _____
   _____
   _____

2. The home health nurse visits a client with heart failure. In reviewing the client's medications, the nurse notes that the client takes the following daily oral medications: digoxin 0.25 mg, furosemide 10 mg, and captopril 0.625 mg. After speaking to the client and wife, the nurse suspects digitalis toxicity. Which question helps the nurse gather more information specific to digitalis toxicity?
   a. "Do you get light-headed when you get out of bed?"
   b. "Do you need to sleep with more than one pillow?"
   c. "Do you have to get up to urinate more frequently?"
   d. "Have you had any nausea, vomiting, or diarrhea?"

   Rationale for your selection: _____
   _____
   _____
   _____

3. The nurse is assigned to a client with heart failure. The nurse's morning lung assessment indicates crackles and wheezes in the mid to lower lung bases, R 32, and the client is restless. Which nursing intervention is of priority initially?
   a. Assess capillary refill.
   b. Take the pulse oximetry.
   c. Limit client activity.
   d. Assess fluid intake.

   Rationale for your selection: _____
   _____
   _____
   _____

ANSWER KEY FOR
APPLYING CRITICAL THINKING SKILLS TO TEST QUESTIONS

HELPFUL HINTS: Read all test questions carefully. Identify key words in the question that will guide you in answering the question. In these test questions the **key words** to consider are **"most indicative," "information specific to,"** and **"priority initially."** Compare your rationale with the one in the test question.

1. The nurse admits a 69-year-old male client with heart failure. The physician orders furosemide 60 mg IVP stat, digoxin 0.25 mg po, and KCl 20 mEq po now. Which assessment finding is most indicative of an ineffective response 2 hours after the administration of all the medications?
   a. Pulse 89, irregular
   b. Urine output 60 mL
   c. Pulse oximetry 94%
   d. Pitting edema in the lower extremities

Rationale: The answer is (b). Although output falls within the parameters of renal function, the client received furosemide IV and diuresis is the desired effect. Options (a), (c), and (d) are expected findings in a client with HF.

2. The home health nurse visits a client with heart failure. In reviewing the client's medications, the nurse notes that the client takes the following daily oral medications: digoxin 0.25 mg, furosemide 10 mg, and captopril 0.625 mg. After speaking to the client and wife, the nurse suspects digitalis toxicity. Which question helps the nurse gather more information specific to digitalis toxicity?
   a. "Do you get light-headed when you get out of bed?"
   b. "Do you need to sleep with more than one pillow?"
   c. "Do you have to get up to urinate more frequently?"
   d. "Have you had any nausea, vomiting, or diarrhea?"

Rationale: The answer is (d). Although these signs and symptoms are frequently seen with all drug therapy, they are frequently early side effects of digitalis toxicity. Options (a), (b), and (c) relate to the action of the other drugs.

3. The nurse is assigned to a client with heart failure. The nurse's morning lung assessment indicates crackles and wheezes in the mid to lower lung bases, R 32, and the client is restless. Which nursing intervention is of priority initially?
   a. Assess capillary refill.
   b. Take the pulse oximetry.
   c. Limit client activity.
   d. Assess fluid intake.

Rationale: The answer is (b). Client assessment indicates rapid breathing and possible hypoxia. To fully assess the respiratory status of the client, it is important to take the pulse oximetry. Options (a), (c), and (d) are important—but not priority—interventions.

2-14 THE PATIENT WITH A STROKE

0700 Handoff Report:

S	Mr. H, 68 years old, experienced a right-sided ischemic stroke. He was admitted to the telemetry unit 2 days ago, and he has been on heparin therapy. Mr. H had a restful night, and there were no changes in his condition. The latest information on the EHR nursing notes indicates: Hand grips R strong, L weak, speech slurred, BP 166/102. He is experiencing short-term memory loss. At 0800 you prepare to assist Mr. H with his breakfast.

The following patient care plan information is available:

VS q4h I & O (✓) Neuro checks q4h Up in chair today O_2 @ 2 L/min/NP Hospital day: #3	IV: 500 mL D5W with heparin 20,000 units infuse at 1000 units/hr via ® subclavian line Foley (✓) care bid ROM to left upper and lower extremities Serum K^+, Na^+, & CBC today PTT q6h (Follow heparin protocol) Dx: Ischemic stroke with left-sided hemiparesis	Diet: Dysphagia (to be determined after swallow evaluation) Swallowing precautions Routine med: Docusate sodium 20 mg (5 mL) po bid

Prioritize the following five **recommended nursing interventions** as you would do them to take care of Mr. H. Write a number in the box to identify the order of your interventions (#1 = first intervention, #2 = second intervention, etc.), and state a **rationale** for each intervention.

INTERVENTIONS	PRIORITY #	RATIONALE
• Sit in high Fowler's position	☐	
• Place food on right side for patient to see	☐	
• Place food into side of mouth that has feeling sensation	☐	
• Check inside of mouth for food caught between gums and teeth (pocketing)	☐	
• Maintain high Fowler's position for 30–45 minutes	☐	

KEY POINTS TO CONSIDER _____

_____

_____

_____

As morning care is given to Mr. H you assess the following:
1. Does not turn head if spoken to from left side
2. Left hand and arm elevated on a pillow
3. Passive range of motion is performed to extremities on the left side
4. Antiembolic stockings on with sequential compression device on
5. Lack of awareness of left side
6. Heparin infusing at 25 mL/hr via pump

Collaborative Learning Activity: With a partner, **do the following: (1) select the one nursing diagnosis** that is a priority at this time, **(2) provide a rationale** for your selection, and **(3) list the nursing interventions** that assist you to meet the needs of the patient.

All of the following nursing diagnoses may apply to Mr. H:

Risk for injury: falls, Deficient knowledge, Fear, Anxiety, Risk for infection, Impaired tissue integrity, Constipation, Impaired swallowing, Impaired verbal communication, Bathing self-care deficit, Impaired urinary elimination, Disturbed body image, Risk for impaired skin integrity, Ineffective peripheral tissue perfusion, Unilateral neglect, Risk for aspiration, Risk for disuse syndrome

Nursing Diagnosis	Rationale	Nursing Interventions

Mr. H's laboratory data are available. The results are as follows: PTT 250 sec (control 38 sec), K$^+$ 3.5 mEq, Na$^+$ 145 mEq, Hgb 11.4 g/dL, Hct 34%, platelets 110,000/mm^3.

Based on **Mr. H's laboratory** data, identify and write the **priority problem** in the box below. Then, starting with the small box labeled **#1, prioritize** the **nursing interventions** for this situation and **identify** your follow-up action plan for Mr. H.

NURSING INTERVENTIONS

A. Notify physician

B. Prepare to administer protamine sulfate (if ordered)

C. Assess for petechiae

D. Monitor urine color

E. Monitor neuro status

F. Take the VS

DECISION-MAKING DIAGRAM

New Action Plan

#1 #2 #3 #4 #5 #6

Priority Problem

NOTES _____

APPLYING CRITICAL THINKING SKILLS TO TEST QUESTIONS

INSTRUCTIONS: Circle the one best answer for each test question. Write your rationale for selecting the answer. To enhance your learning and test-taking skills, discuss your answer and rationale with a partner. The answer and the rationale can be found on the back of this page.

1. The nurse is caring for a client who had a right-sided stroke 5 days ago and is experiencing unilateral neglect. In delegating the care of the client, which nursing intervention is of priority? The nurse instructs the nursing assistant to
   a. have the client use a communication board.
   b. place the food tray to the right side of the body.
   c. remind the client to look at the left side of the body.
   d. provide passive range of motion to the left side of the body.

   Rationale for your selection: _____
   _____
   _____
   _____

2. The nurse walks into a client's room. The client is in supine position and the wife is stroking his hand. The client had a left-sided stroke 7 days ago, just took 30% of the dysphagic diet, and has an indwelling urinary catheter. Which nursing action is of priority for this client?
   a. Raise the head of the bed.
   b. Encourage the wife to talk softly to the client.
   c. Remind the client to look at and touch the affected side.
   d. Assess the color and amount of output.

   Rationale for your selection: _____
   _____
   _____
   _____

3. The nurse is preparing to administer oral medications to a client who is on a dysphagic diet. Which nursing action is best in administering the 0900 medication to the client? Crush the medication and
   a. put the crushed medication in 15 mL of tap water.
   b. mix the crushed medication in 4 ounces of applesauce.
   c. dissolve the crushed medication in 30 mL of warm water.
   d. mix the crushed medication in 30 mL of thickened liquid.

   Rationale for your selection: _____
   _____
   _____
   _____

2 Priority Setting and Decision Making

ANSWER KEY FOR
APPLYING CRITICAL THINKING SKILLS TO TEST QUESTIONS

HELPFUL HINTS: Read all test questions carefully. Identify key words in the question that will guide you in answering the question. In these test questions the **key words** to consider are **"priority"** and **"best."** Compare your rationale with the one in the test question.

1. The nurse is caring for a client who had a right-sided stroke 5 days ago and is experiencing unilateral neglect. In delegating the care of the client, which nursing intervention is of priority? The nurse instructs the nursing assistant to
   a. have the client use a communication board.
   b. place the food tray to the right side of the body.
   c. remind the client to look at the left side of the body.
   d. provide passive range of motion to the left side of the body.

   Rationale: The answer is (c). Clients who have a right-sided stroke have spatial and perceptual deficits. Clients will neglect the left side of the body. Options (a), (b), and (d) do not correlate the clients need to the intervention.

2. The nurse walks into a client's room. The client is in supine position and the wife is stroking his hand. The client had a left-sided stroke 7 days ago, just took 30% of the dysphagic diet, and has an indwelling urinary catheter. Which nursing action is of priority for this client?
   a. Raise the head of the bed.
   b. Encourage the wife to talk softly to the client.
   c. Remind the client to look at and touch the affected side.
   d. Assess the color and amount of output.

   Rationale: The answer is (a). After eating, the client should remain in Fowler's position to prevent aspiration. Options (b), (c), and (d) are important, but they are not priorities at this time.

3. The nurse is preparing to administer oral medications to a client who is on a dysphagic diet. Which nursing action is best in administering the 0900 medication to the client? Crush the medication and
   a. put the crushed medication in 15 mL of tap water.
   b. mix the crushed medication in 4 ounces of applesauce.
   c. dissolve the crushed medication in 30 mL of warm water.
   d. mix the crushed medication in 30 mL of thickened liquid.

   Rationale: The answer is (d). Use a small amount of thickened liquid to mix and administer the medications. Options (a) and (c) are not appropriate because water may cause the client to aspirate. Option (b) is mixing the medications in too large a quantity of applesauce.

2-15 THE PATIENT WITH CHRONIC OBSTRUCTIVE PULMONARY DISEASE

0700 Handoff Report:

S	Mr. Y, a 66-year-old man, was admitted with exacerbation of his chronic obstructive pulmonary disease (COPD). He has been agitated during the night and is dyspneic this morning. The 0600 vital signs are T 98.8°F, P 102, R 32, BP 146/98, pain level 0–1, pulse ox was 89% (room air). He has an IV of D5W infusing at 75 mL/hr. Oxygen was started at 2 L/min/nasal cannula and the pulse ox is up to 90%. He receives albuterol inhaler 2 puffs q4h prn and salmeterol (Serevent) inhaler 2 puffs q12h with spacer device and prednisone 20 mg po daily.
B	The patient has a 40-year history of smoking. He has noticed an increase in sputum production and SOB for the last 2 weeks. Rapid and shallow breathing and use of accessory respiratory muscles were present on admission.
A	Respirations short and shallow, pursed-lip breathing noted. Oxygen at 2 L/min/nasal cannula. Skin cool, 1+ pitting edema noted in bilateral lower extremities, pedal pulses present, weak.
R	The following nursing interventions are recommended initially:

Prioritize the following five **recommended nursing interventions** as you would do them to initially take care of Mr. Y. Write a number in the box to identify the order of your interventions (#1 = first intervention, #2 = second intervention, etc.), and state a **rationale** for each intervention.

INTERVENTIONS	PRIORITY #	RATIONALE
• Auscultate lung sounds	☐	_____
• Assess pulse oximeter, oxygen, and nasal cannula	☐	_____
• Retake the vital signs	☐	_____
• Administer salmeterol inhaler using spacer device	☐	_____
• Place in high Fowler's position	☐	_____

KEY POINTS TO CONSIDER _____

_____

_____

As you provide morning care to Mr. Y you assess the following signs and symptoms:
1. Nonproductive cough; long expiratory phase during respiration
2. Increased shortness of breath with mild exertion
3. Crackles audible throughout the bilateral lung fields
4. Anxious and restless

Collaborative Learning Activity: With a partner, **do the following: (1) select the one nursing diagnosis** that is a priority at this time, **(2) provide a rationale** for your selection, and **(3) list the nursing interventions** that assist you to meet the needs of the patient.

All of the following nursing diagnoses may apply to Mr. Y:

Ineffective breathing pattern, Ineffective airway clearance, Risk for injury, Risk for infection, Anxiety, Impaired gas exchange, Activity intolerance, Risk for impaired skin integrity, Imbalanced nutrition: less than body requirements, Sexual dysfunction

Nursing Diagnosis	Rationale	Nursing Interventions

At **12:00 noon** the patient care assistant reports that Mr. Y is very warm and that his VS are T 102°F, P 98, R 32, BP 140/84. He is expectorating thick yellow-colored sputum.

Based on the situation at **12:00 noon**, identify and write the **priority problem** in the box below. Then, starting with the small box labeled **#1, prioritize** the **nursing interventions** for this situation and **identify** your follow-up action plan for Mr. Y.

NURSING INTERVENTIONS

DECISION-MAKING DIAGRAM

A. Auscultate lung sounds

B. Administer antipyretic if ordered

C. Assess orientation and LOC

D. Check oxygen saturation level

E. Retake VS in 2 hours

F. Inform physician

New Action Plan

#1 #2 #3 #4 #5 #6

Priority Problem

NOTES _____

_____

APPLYING CRITICAL THINKING SKILLS TO TEST QUESTIONS

INSTRUCTIONS: Circle the one best answer for each test question. Write your rationale for selecting the answer. To enhance your learning and test-taking skills, discuss your answer and rationale with a partner. The answer and the rationale can be found on the back of this page.

1. The nurse is caring for a client who was admitted with an exacerbation of COPD. The client's respirations are 28 with dyspnea on exertion. The client is receiving 2 L/min of oxygen per nasal cannula. The morning pulse oximetry is 92%. Which nursing intervention is of priority?
   a. Monitor the client.
   b. Notify the physician.
   c. Get an order to increase the oxygen.
   d. Place in semi-Fowler's position.

   Rationale for your selection: _____
   _____
   _____
   _____

2. The client has a long history of COPD and is currently experiencing an exacerbation of COPD. The following lab work is done this morning: complete blood cell count, arterial blood gases, and an electrolyte panel consisting of K^+, Na^+, Cl^-, carbon dioxide, blood urea nitrogen, and fasting blood glucose. Which laboratory data will require immediate follow-up?
   a. PaO_2 WNL
   b. Increased RBCs
   c. Increased $Paco_2$
   d. Hgb WNL

   Rationale for your selection: _____
   _____
   _____
   _____

3. The client is admitted with an acute exacerbation of COPD. Which assessment finding is most indicative of a potential complication?
   a. R 32, increasingly anxious and restless
   b. Using accessory muscles during respiration
   c. Pulse oximetry 92%, pursed-lip breathing
   d. Expectorating copious amount of white phlegm

   Rationale for your selection: _____
   _____
   _____
   _____

ANSWER KEY FOR
APPLYING CRITICAL THINKING SKILLS TO TEST QUESTIONS

HELPFUL HINTS: Read all test questions carefully. Identify key words in the question that will guide you in answering the question. In these test questions the **key words** to consider are **"priority," "immediate,"** and **"most indicative."** Compare your rationale with the one in the test question.

1. The nurse is caring for a client who was admitted with an exacerbation of COPD. The client's respirations are 28 with dyspnea on exertion. The client is receiving 2 L/min of oxygen per nasal cannula. The morning pulse oximetry is 92%. Which nursing intervention is of priority?
   a. Monitor the client.
   b. Notify the physician.
   c. Get an order to increase the oxygen.
   d. Place in semi-Fowler's position.

Rationale: The answer is (a). The client is manifesting signs and symptoms consistent with COPD. Clients with COPD have some degree of hypoxia. Options (b) and (c) are not appropriate at this time. Option (d) is not the best position for a client with COPD.

2. The client has a long history of COPD and is currently experiencing an exacerbation of COPD. The following lab work is done this morning: complete blood cell count, arterial blood gases, and an electrolyte panel consisting of K^+, Na^+, Cl^-, carbon dioxide, blood urea nitrogen, and fasting blood glucose. Which laboratory data will require immediate follow-up?
   a. PaO_2 WNL
   b. Increased RBCs
   c. Increased $Paco_2$
   d. Hgb WNL

Rationale: The answer is (a). Hypoxemia provides the stimulus for the respiratory drive in clients with COPD. Increased oxygen levels may depress the respiratory drive. Options (b) and (c) are expected findings. Option (d) does not require immediate follow-up.

3. The client is admitted with an acute exacerbation of COPD. Which assessment finding is most indicative of a potential complication?
   a. R 32, increasingly anxious and restless
   b. Using accessory muscles during respiration
   c. Pulse oximetry 92%, pursed-lip breathing
   d. Expectorating copious amount of white phlegm

Rationale: The answer is (a). Increasing anxiousness and restlessness are signs indicating hypoxemia. Options (b), (c), and (d) are expected findings for a client with an exacerbation of COPD.

2-16 THE PATIENT WITH A CHEST TUBE

0700 Handoff Report:

 Mr. G, 23 years old, has been in the hospital for 2 days after being stabbed in the chest. He has a posterior chest tube connected to a Pleur-evac system. He had a restful night. Pain level 2. Chest tube drainage was 15 mL. Midnight VS were T 99°F, P 90, R 22, BP 128/74, and the pulse ox at 4:00 AM was 95%. He is on O2 @ 3 L/min/NP.

The following patient care plan information is available:

VS q4h I & O (✓) Pulse ox q4h Amb with assist prn O$_2$ @ 3 L/min/NP Chest tube to low con't suction	IV: D5/0.45% NaCl q12h IVPB: cefazolin 1 g q6h Chest x-ray today ABG today Code status: Full	Diet: Soft Routine med: Docusate sodium 100 mg caps i po daily

Prioritize the following five **recommended nursing interventions** as you would do them to take care of Mr. G. Write a number in the box to identify the order of your interventions (#1 = first intervention, #2 = second intervention, etc.), and state a **rationale** for each intervention.

INTERVENTIONS	PRIORITY #	RATIONALE
• Check the pulse oximetry	☐	_____
• Assess for fluctuation in the water-seal chamber and bubbling in the suction-control chamber	☐	_____
• Check for the previous shift's fluid level marking on the tape	☐	_____
• Assess chest tube patency and drainage	☐	_____
• Ask Mr. G to cough and deep breathe	☐	_____

KEY POINTS TO CONSIDER _____

_____

_____

After breakfast, Mr. G is transported to the x-ray department by wheelchair. On his return to his room you assess the following:
1. VS: T 99.8°F, P 102, R 26, BP 132/90
2. Complains of dyspnea, crackles auscultated, anxious
3. Oxygen off, oxygen saturation at 88%

Collaborative Learning Activity: With a partner, **do the following: (1) select the one nursing diagnosis** that is a priority at this time, **(2) provide a rationale** for your selection, and **(3) list the nursing interventions** that assist you to meet the needs of the patient.

All of the following nursing diagnoses may apply to Mr. G:

Ineffective airway clearance, Ineffective breathing pattern, Impaired gas exchange, Risk for injury, Deficient knowledge, Fear, Anxiety, Risk for infection, Impaired tissue integrity

Nursing Diagnosis	Rationale	Nursing Interventions

One hour later, Mr. G becomes increasingly restless and, as you take his VS, he abruptly moves and the chest tube is pulled out.

On the basis of the situation **1 hour later,** identify and write the **priority problem** in the box below. Then, starting with the small box labeled **#1, prioritize** the **nursing interventions** for this situation and **identify** your follow-up action plan for Mr. G.

NURSING INTERVENTIONS

A. Instruct Mr. G to take a deep breath and hold

B. Cover chest tube site with occlusive dressing

C. Apply gloves if possible

D. Maintain oxygen @ 3 L/min/NP

E. Notify physician

F. Pinch chest tube site together

DECISION-MAKING DIAGRAM

New Action Plan

#1   #2   #3   #4   #5   #6

Priority Problem

NOTES _____

_____

APPLYING CRITICAL THINKING SKILLS TO TEST QUESTIONS

INSTRUCTIONS: Circle the one best answer for each test question. Write your rationale for selecting the answer. To enhance your learning and test-taking skills, discuss your answer and rationale with a partner. The answer and the rationale can be found on the back of this page.

1. The nurse is preparing to assist with the insertion of a chest tube that will be attached to a closed-chest drainage system without suction. In monitoring the closed-chest drainage system, the nurse would expect to initially assess for
   a. fluctuation of water in the water-seal chamber during respirations.
   b. constant fluid fluctuations in the drainage-collection chamber.
   c. continuous bubbling in the suction-control chamber.
   d. occasional bubbling in the suction-control chamber.

   Rationale for your selection: _____
   _____
   _____
   _____

2. The client has a chest tube connected to a closed-chest drainage system attached to suction and is being prepared to transfer to another room on a stretcher. To safely transport the client, it is most important for the nurse to
   a. clamp the chest tube during the transport.
   b. get portable suction equipment before transferring the client.
   c. keep the closed-chest drainage system below the level of the chest.
   d. place the closed-chest drainage system next to the client on the stretcher.

   Rationale for your selection: _____
   _____
   _____
   _____

3. The physician is preparing to remove the client's chest tube. Just before removing the chest tube, the physician tells the client to take a deep breath and hold it. The intervention is primarily done to
   a. distract the patient while the chest tube is removed.
   b. minimize the negative pressure within the pleural space.
   c. decrease the degree of discomfort to the client.
   d. increase the intrathoracic pressure temporarily during removal.

   Rationale for your selection: _____
   _____
   _____
   _____

ANSWER KEY FOR
APPLYING CRITICAL THINKING SKILLS TO TEST QUESTIONS

HELPFUL HINTS: Read all test questions carefully. Identify key words in the question that will guide you in answering the question. In these test questions the **key words** to consider are **"initially," "most important,"** and **"primarily."** Compare your rationale with the one in the test question.

1. The nurse is preparing to assist with the insertion of a chest tube that will be attached to a closed-chest drainage system without suction. In monitoring the closed-chest drainage system, the nurse would expect to initially assess for
   a. fluctuation of water in the water-seal chamber during respirations.
   b. constant fluid fluctuations in the drainage-collection chamber.
   c. continuous bubbling in the suction-control chamber.
   d. occasional bubbling in the suction-control chamber.

   Rationale: The answer is (a). Fluctuations of water during inspiration and expiration in the water-seal chamber indicate normal functioning. Option (b) should not be seen in the collection chamber. Options (c) and (d) should not be seen because suction has not been applied to the suction-control chamber.

2. The client has a chest tube connected to a closed-chest drainage system attached to suction and is being prepared to transfer to another room on a stretcher. To safely transport the client, it is most important for the nurse to
   a. clamp the chest tube during the transport.
   b. get portable suction equipment before transferring the client.
   c. keep the closed-chest drainage system below the level of the chest.
   d. place the closed-chest drainage system next to the client on the stretcher.

   Rationale: The answer is (c). Keeping the closed-chest drainage system below the level of the chest allows for continuous drainage and prevents any backflow pressure. Options (a) and (d) should not be done because they will increase pressure in the pleural space. Option (b) is not the most important.

3. The physician is preparing to remove the client's chest tube. Just before removing the chest tube, the physician tells the client to take a deep breath and hold it. The intervention is primarily done to
   a. distract the patient while the chest tube is removed.
   b. minimize the negative pressure within the pleural space.
   c. decrease the degree of discomfort to the client.
   d. increase the intrathoracic pressure temporarily during removal.

   Rationale: The answer is (d). This is done to decrease the risk of atmospheric air entering the pleural space during removal. Options (a) and (c) are not the primary reasons for this intervention. Option (b) is not correct because negative pressure is desired within the lung.

2-17 THE PATIENT WITH UROSEPSIS

1500 Handoff Report:

S	Mr. TD, 79 years old, was admitted today to the hospital with the diagnosis of urosepsis. He has an IV of lactated Ringer's infusing at 100 mL/hr. Ceftriaxone 1 g IVPB qAM is ordered. He is on I & O q8h, soft diet, bathroom privileges with assistance, and acetaminophen 500 mg tabs i po q4h for temperature greater than 38°C. His 2:00 PM VS were T 38°C, P 78, R 22, BP 146/88, pulse ox 96%. He has been more restless this afternoon, trying to get out of bed and disoriented to time and place. His urine is dark yellow and cloudy. He was moved closer to the nurse's station to assist with frequent monitoring.
B	Mr. TD lives alone. His daughter took him to the doctor when she visited him and found that he had a fever and he complained of frequent urination and incontinence. His oral intake has been minimal.
A	The certified nurse assistant reports to you the change of shift VS of T 38.8°C, P 88, R 24, BP 144/80, pulse ox 97%.
R	The following nursing interventions are recommended initially:

Prioritize the following five **recommended nursing interventions** as you, the nurse, would do them to initially take care of Mr. TD. Write a number in the box to identify the order of your interventions (#1 = first intervention, #2 = second intervention, etc.), and state a **rationale** for each intervention.

Interventions	Priority #	Rationale
• Assess for bed alarm/safety features	☐	_____
• Administer acetaminophen 500 mg tabs i	☐	_____
• Gather urinary output data	☐	_____
• Assess mental status	☐	_____
• Perform a body systems physical assessment	☐	_____

KEY POINTS TO CONSIDER _____

_____

_____

Priority Setting and Decision Making

You perform a follow-up assessment at 7:00 PM and assess the following:
1. VS: T 38.5°C, P 98, R 22, BP 120/76, pulse ox 94%
2. Fine crackles audible on auscultation in the bilateral lower lung fields
3. He is sleepy, lethargic
4. He was incontinent of a scant amount of urine

Collaborative Learning Activity: With a partner, **do the following: (1) select** the **one nursing diagnosis** that is a priority at this time, **(2) provide a rationale** for your selection, and **(3) list the nursing interventions** that assist you to meet the needs of the patient.

All of the following nursing diagnoses may apply to Mr. TD:

Risk for impaired skin integrity, Impaired urinary elimination, Risk for injury, Acute confusion, Hyperthermia, Deficient fluid volume, Imbalanced nutrition: less than body requirements, Risk for shock, Ineffective breathing pattern, Fatigue

Nursing Diagnosis	Rationale	Nursing Interventions

As you take his **8:00 PM** vital signs, you assess the following signs and symptoms: Lethargic, skin very warm and flushed, VS: T 39.1°C, P 130, R 28, BP 90/54, pulse ox 88%.

Based on the situation at **8:00 PM,** identify and write the **priority problem** in the box below. Then, starting with the small box labeled **#1, prioritize** the **nursing interventions** for this situation and **identify** your follow-up action plan for Mr. TD.

NURSING INTERVENTIONS

A. Check pulse ox

B. Prepare to start O_2

C. Prepare to insert indwelling urinary catheter

D. Take vital signs q5min

E. Record findings

F. Notify physician

DECISION-MAKING DIAGRAM

New Action Plan

#1 #2 #3 #4 #5 #6

Priority Problem

NOTES _____

2-18 THE PATIENT WITH A TRANSURETHRAL RESECTION OF THE PROSTATE

1200 PACU Transfer Handoff Report:

S Mr. J, 68 years old, had a TURP this morning. His vital signs have been stable. He is sleepy but easily arousable. The 3-way urinary catheter is taped to his thigh and the urinary drainage bag was emptied at 1130 prior to transfer, and his vital signs at that time were T 98.2°F, P 88, R 20, BP 150/88, pulse ox 98%. The normal saline irrigation bag is infusing since there were some small clots in the urine output; there is 200 mL left in the irrigation bag. The IV is infusing at 100 mL/hr, 500 mL are left.

The following post of orders are on the patient care plan below:

VS q4h I & O qs Antiembolic hose Sequential teds ×24 hrs Up in chair this PM	IV: lactated Ringer's @100 mL/hr IV site: RFA # 20 g 3-way urinary catheter to gravity with continuous irrigation of NS to keep UA free of clots Dx: Benign prostatic hypertrophy	Diet: Clear liquids this PM PRN medication: B & O supp. q4h prn bladder spasms

At 1230, Mr. J is alert, and you notice that his urinary drainage bag contains dark red urine and some blood clots; the normal saline solution irrigation bag is empty. Mr. J is complaining of having the urge to void.

Prioritize the following five **recommended nursing interventions** as you would do them to take care of Mr. J. Write a number in the box to identify the order of your interventions (#1 = first intervention, #2 = second intervention, etc.), and state a **rationale** for each intervention.

INTERVENTIONS	PRIORITY #	RATIONALE
• Take VS, assess pain level	☐	_____
• Assess continuous urinary irrigation system	☐	_____
• Address patient's complaint of "having the urge to void"	☐	_____
• Perform a body systems physical assessment	☐	_____
• Hang up new normal saline solution irrigation bag	☐	_____

KEY POINTS TO CONSIDER _____

On the first postop day you assess the following on Mr. J:
1. VS: T 99.6°F, P 98, R 24, BP 154/90, pulse ox 96
2. Urinary catheter taped to thigh, urine pinkish, no clots
3. Grimaces and says, "I didn't think it would be this tough." States pain level 8 out of 10.
4. Further states, "I do not think sex will ever be the same."

Collaborative Learning Activity: With a partner, **do the following: (1) select** the **one nursing diagnosis** that is a priority at this time, **(2) provide a rationale** for your selection, and **(3) list the nursing interventions** that assist you to meet the needs of the patient.

All of the following nursing diagnoses may apply to Mr. J:

Risk for infection, Impaired tissue integrity, Excess fluid volume, Deficient knowledge, Anxiety, Risk for injury, Impaired urinary elimination, Acute pain, Ineffective sexuality pattern, Situational low self-esteem, Urinary retention, Risk for bleeding

Nursing Diagnosis	Rationale	Nursing Interventions

The normal saline solution irrigation is discontinued at 12:00 noon the first postop day. Toward the end of the shift **(3:00 PM),** you **assess** the following on Mr. J: complaints of pain, states pain level 10, no output since 12:00 PM, abdominal distention, and Mr. J is restless.

On the basis of the **3:00 PM assessment,** identify and write the **priority problem** in the box below. Then, starting with the small box labeled **#1, prioritize** the **nursing interventions** for this situation and **identify** your follow-up action plan for Mr. J.

NURSING INTERVENTIONS

A. Take the vital signs

B. Inform MD

C. Prepare to do a urinary irrigation

D. Give an antispasmodic

E. Place in low Fowler's to semi-Fowler's position

F. Encourage fluids

DECISION-MAKING DIAGRAM

New Action Plan

#1 #2 #3 #4 #5 #6

Priority Problem

NOTES _____

APPLYING CRITICAL THINKING SKILLS TO TEST QUESTIONS

INSTRUCTIONS: Circle the one best answer for each test question. Write your rationale for selecting the answer. To enhance your learning and test-taking skills, discuss your answer and rationale with a partner. The answer and the rationale can be found on the back of this page.

1. The client is 1 day postop TURP. He has a three-way indwelling urinary catheter with continuous bladder irrigation. During handoff report, the nurse learns that the client's output was 1700 mL. A priority nursing intervention is for the nurse to
   a. check the client's oral and parenteral intake for the previous shift.
   b. know the amount of irrigation fluid that infused during the previous shift.
   c. assess if the client has passed any urinary clots through the catheter.
   d. ensure that the urinary output is yellow to pinkish in color.

   Rationale for your selection: _____
   _____
   _____
   _____

2. The physician orders continuous bladder irrigation for a client who had a TURP this morning. To effectively implement this order, it is most important for the nurse to infuse the irrigation solution
   a. to maintain urine output clear to light pink in color.
   b. when the urine is red with visible clots.
   c. so that the intake equals the output.
   d. at a rate of 50 mL/hr.

   Rationale for your selection: _____
   _____
   _____
   _____

3. The client is 2 days postop TURP and is complaining of an increasing urge to void. The client has a three-way urinary catheter with continuous bladder irrigation. After assessing that the catheter is patent and is draining freely, the priority nursing intervention is to
   a. reassure the client that the catheter is draining appropriately.
   b. document the client's complaints and assessment findings.
   c. give the client antispasmodic medication.
   d. notify the physician.

   Rationale for your selection: _____
   _____
   _____
   _____

ANSWER KEY FOR
APPLYING CRITICAL THINKING SKILLS TO TEST QUESTIONS

HELPFUL HINTS: Read all test questions carefully. Identify key words in the question that will guide you in answering the question. In these test questions the **key words** to consider are **"priority"** and **"most important."** Compare your rationale with the one in the test question.

1. The client is 1 day postop TURP. He has a three-way indwelling urinary catheter with continuous bladder irrigation. During handoff report, the nurse learns that the client's output was 1700 mL. A priority nursing intervention is for the nurse to
   a. check the client's oral and parenteral intake for the previous shift.
   b. know the amount of irrigation fluid that infused during the previous shift.
   c. assess if the client has passed any urinary clots through the catheter.
   d. ensure that the urinary output is yellow to pinkish in color.

Rationale: The answer is (b). It is important to know the amount of irrigation solution that infused to assess the actual urinary output. Options (a), (c), and (d) are good interventions but not of priority.

2. The physician orders continuous bladder irrigation for a client who had a TURP this morning. To effectively implement this order, it is most important for the nurse to infuse the irrigation solution
   a. to maintain urine output clear to light pink in color.
   b. when the urine is red with visible clots.
   c. so that the intake equals the output.
   d. at a rate of 50 mL/hr.

Rationale: The answer is (a). Continuous irrigation is given to prevent clot formation and prevent obstruction of the catheter. Options (b), (c), and (d) are not appropriate interventions.

3. The client is 2 days postop TURP and is complaining of an increasing urge to void. The client has a three-way urinary catheter with continuous bladder irrigation. After assessing that the catheter is patent and is draining freely, the priority nursing intervention is to
   a. reassure the client that the catheter is draining appropriately.
   b. document the client's complaints and assessment findings.
   c. give the client antispasmodic medication.
   d. notify the physician.

Rationale: The answer is (c). Bladder spasms can cause the client to feel an urge to void. Options (a) and (b) do not address the client's current need. Option (d) is not appropriate at this time.

2-19 THE PATIENT RECEIVING A BLOOD TRANSFUSION

0700 Handoff Report:

> **S** Mr. TA, 34 years old, was admitted after a motor vehicle accident: pedestrian versus car. He sustained multiple injuries throughout his body. He will receive 2 units of whole blood this morning. He has NS 0.9% infusing at TKO rate through a Y-type blood administration set and has a 19-gauge cannula in the RFA. The MD obtains the consent form and orders to infuse each unit over 3 hours. As you get out of the report, the lab notifies you that the first unit of blood is ready.

Prioritize the following five **recommended nursing interventions** as you would do them to take care of Mr. TA. Write a number in the box to identify the order of your interventions (#1 = first intervention, #2 = second intervention, etc.), and state a **rationale** for each intervention.

INTERVENTIONS	PRIORITY #	RATIONALE
• Take an initial set of vital signs, assess pain level, pulse ox	☐	
• Obtain the blood from the lab	☐	
• Assess the IV site	☐	
• Start the transfusion	☐	
⚠ • Verify MD order, blood compatibility, and patient ID with another licensed staff nurse at patient bedside (point of care patient identification)	☐	

KEY POINTS TO CONSIDER _____

_____

_____

_____

Priority Setting and Decision Making — 2

You assess the following during the start of the transfusion on Mr. TA:

1. VS: T 97.6°F, P 80, R 18, BP 136/78 (pretransfusion)
2. VS: T 98.2°F, P 90, R 22, BP 130/70 (15 minutes after the start of the transfusion)
3. No complaints of itching, hives, SOB,
4. Transfusion rate increased to 100 mL/hr

Collaborative Learning Activity: With a partner, **do the following: (1) select** the **one nursing diagnosis** that is a priority at this time, **(2) provide a rationale** for your selection, and **(3) list the nursing interventions** that assist you to meet the needs of the patient.

All of the following nursing diagnoses may apply to Mr. TA:

Risk for infection, Fatigue, Risk for impaired skin integrity, Deficient fluid volume, Deficient knowledge, Anxiety, Risk for injury, Acute pain

Nursing Diagnosis	Rationale	Nursing Interventions

After 20 minutes, Mr. TA's **assessment** includes: Skin flushed, P 120, R 32, BP 100/60, complains of chest pain and chills.

Based on the above **assessment,** identify and write the **priority problem** in the box below. Then, starting with the small box labeled **#1, prioritize** the **nursing interventions** for this situation and **identify** your follow-up action plan for Mr. TA.

NURSING INTERVENTIONS　　　　**DECISION-MAKING DIAGRAM**

A. Stop the transfusion

B. Inform MD/Lab

C. Save the next voided specimen

D. Start 0.9% NS at TKO rate with new IV tubing

E. Take VS, pulse ox

F. Save the transfusion unit

New Action Plan

#1　#2　#3　#4　#5　#6

□　□　□　□　□　□

Priority Problem

NOTES _____

_____

2-20 THE PATIENT WITH NEUTROPENIA

0700 Handoff Report:

S	Mrs. K, 68 years old, was admitted 2 days ago with neutropenia. She had outpatient chemotherapy treatment 7 days ago. Her absolute neutrophil count (ANC) is 500 cells/mm^3. Her 0600 VS are T 98.8°F, P 90, R 22, BP 122/72, pulse ox 98%, pain level 0.

The following patient care plan information is available:

VS q4h I & O (✓) Protective isolation precautions (✓) CBC with diff—today Chest x-ray done	Diet: ↑ protein, ↑ calorie (no raw vegetables/fresh fruit) IV: D5W @ 125 mL/hr IV site: RFA (inserted 2 days ago) Code status: Full	Routine medication: Docusate sodium 100 mg po daily 0900 PRN medication: Acetaminophen 325 tabs ii q4h po prn for temp greater than 100.4°F

Prioritize the following five **recommended nursing interventions** as you would do them to take care of Mrs. K. Write a number in the box to identify the order of your interventions (#1 = first intervention, #2 = second intervention, etc.), and state a **rationale** for each intervention.

INTERVENTIONS	PRIORITY #	RATIONALE
• Wash hands	☐	_____
• Assess the IV site	☐	_____
• Provide fresh water at bedside	☐	_____
• Assess oral mucosa	☐	_____
• Take the vital signs, assess pain level, pulse ox	☐	_____

KEY POINTS TO CONSIDER _____

_____

Mrs. K is diagnosed with acute leukemia. Your follow-up assessment includes:
1. Hgb 9.8 g/dL, hematocrit 29%
2. White blood cell count 900/mm³ with an absolute neutrophil count (ANC) 600 cells/µL
3. Monitoring temperature, oral mucosa
4. Platelet count 100,000/mm³

Collaborative Learning Activity: With a partner, **do the following: (1) select the one nursing diagnosis** that is a priority at this time, **(2) provide a rationale** for your selection, and **(3) list the nursing interventions** that assist you to meet the needs of the patient.

All of the following nursing diagnoses may apply to Mrs. K:

Risk for infection, Fatigue, Imbalanced nutrition: less than body requirements, Deficient knowledge, Anxiety, Risk for injury, Impaired oral mucous membrane, Activity intolerance, Risk for impaired skin integrity, Social isolation, Fear, Hopelessness, Impaired physical mobility

Nursing Diagnosis	Rationale	Nursing Interventions

The following day, Mrs. K's **assessment findings** are significant for: Platelet count 30,000/mm³, bleeding time prolonged, oral petechiae, hemoptysis, tachypnea, dyspnea, and a current nosebleed.

On the basis of the most current **assessment,** identify and write the **priority problem** in the box below. Then, starting with the small box labeled **#1, prioritize** the **nursing interventions** for this situation and **identify** your follow-up action plan for Mrs. K.

NURSING INTERVENTIONS

A. Take the vital signs

B. Assess for signs and symptoms of bleeding

C. Assess neurologic status

D. Place in high Fowler's position

E. Pinch nostrils shut; have patient mouth breathe

F. Inform physician

DECISION-MAKING DIAGRAM

New Action Plan

#1 #2 #3 #4 #5 #6

Priority Problem

NOTES _____

2-21 THE PATIENT WITH A HIP FRACTURE

0700 Handoff Report:

Priority Setting and Decision Making

S	Mrs. T, 72 years old, had an open reduction with internal fixation (ORIF) of her right hip yesterday. This is her first postop day. Her right hip dressing has a small amount of dried dark red drainage. She has an IV of D5/0.45% NaCl at 75 mL/hr, oxygen at 2 L/min/nasal cannula, and is on a clear liquid diet. The right leg is warm, pedal pulse present, capillary refill around 2 seconds. IV PCA with morphine sulfate delivering 1 mg/hr continuous infusion. The following medications are ordered: $FeSO_4$ 325 mg po tid with meals, docusate sodium 100 mg po daily. The urinary catheter is draining clear urine and is to be discontinued today. 0600 vital signs are P 80, R 18, BP 110/84, pulse ox 96%, pain level difficult to assess since she is restless and confused this morning.
B	Mrs. T fell at home and sustained a fracture of the right hip. She was brought to the ER by ambulance. She was alert and oriented on admission. After the initial workup, she was taken to surgery.
A	Restless, grabbing linens and moaning. Confused to time and place this morning. Skin warm, IV site patent, O_2 at 2 L/NC. Side rails up.
R	The following nursing interventions are recommended:

Prioritize the following five **recommended nursing interventions** according to Mrs. T's current needs. Write a number in the box to identify the order of your interventions (#1 = first intervention, #2 = second intervention, etc.), and state a **rationale** for each intervention.

INTERVENTIONS	PRIORITY #	RATIONALE
• Assess surgical dressing	☐	
• Take VS, assess pain level, check pulse ox	☐	
• Assess neuro status	☐	
• Assess right leg position and body alignment	☐	
• Check neurovascular status of right leg (CMST)	☐	

KEY POINTS TO CONSIDER _____

During the follow-up assessment for the **first postop day,** you assess the following:
1. Pedal pulse present; weak in the right foot, stronger in left foot
2. Hemoglobin 10.5 g/dL and hematocrit 32%
3. Bowel sounds hypoactive in all quadrants
4. Crackles in the lower bases of the lung

Collaborative Learning Activity: With a partner, **do the following: (1) select the one nursing diagnosis** that is a priority at this time, **(2) provide a rationale** for your selection, and **(3) list the nursing interventions** that assist you to meet the needs of the patient.

All of the following nursing diagnoses may apply to Mrs. T:

Acute pain, Risk for infection, Risk for impaired skin integrity, Impaired urinary elimination, Impaired gas exchange, Fatigue, Impaired physical mobility, Ineffective peripheral tissue perfusion, Acute confusion, Constipation

Nursing Diagnosis	Rationale	Nursing Interventions

On the second postop day Mrs. T is still very confused and is trying to get out of bed. She has bilateral scattered crackles in the lungs, labored breathing, shortness of breath on exertion, R 32, P 108, pulse ox 92%, a productive cough, and whitish sputum. Skin cool, pallor.

Based on the most current situation, identify and write the **priority problem** in the box below. Then, starting with the small box labeled **#1, prioritize** the **nursing interventions** for this situation and **identify** your plan for follow-up care for Mrs. T.

NURSING INTERVENTIONS

A. Monitor P, R, BP q5min

B. Check oxygen saturation continuously

C. Stay with patient

D. Administer O_2 per nasal cannula

E. Call physician

F. Prepare to transfer patient

DECISION-MAKING DIAGRAM

New Action Plan

#1 #2 #3 #4 #5 #6

Priority Problem

NOTES _____

APPLYING CRITICAL THINKING SKILLS TO TEST QUESTIONS

INSTRUCTIONS: Circle the one best answer for each test question. Write your rationale for selecting the answer. To enhance your learning and test-taking skills, discuss your answer and rationale with a partner. The answer and the rationale can be found on the back of this page.

1. The nurse is caring for an 82-year-old client who is 1 day postop left hip replacement. The client has a primary IV infusing at 100 mL/hr, a patient-controlled analgesic device, and a urinary catheter. After assessing the client, the nurse determines that the client is pleasant and cooperative but forgetful. In the afternoon, the nurse notes that the client has become increasingly restless. It is most important for the nurse to
   a. apply a vest restraint.
   b. notify the physician.
   c. check the patient-controlled analgesic device.
   d. assess the client's medical history for dementia.

   Rationale for your selection: _____
   _____
   _____
   _____

2. The nurse is delegating the care of a 79-year-old client 2 days postop hip replacement to a nursing assistant who routinely works on a medical unit. Which instruction given to the nursing assistant is of priority initially?
   a. Have the client cough and deep breathe q2h.
   b. Total the intake and output at 1400.
   c. Use a fracture bedpan for toileting needs.
   d. Wash the client's skin with a mild soap.

   Rationale for your selection: _____
   _____
   _____
   _____

3. The nurse is assisting a client to get out of a chair after having a right hip replacement 3 days ago. The client suddenly complains of pain and tells the nurse that it hurts too much to walk. Which nursing intervention is of priority?
   a. Encourage the client to put most of the weight on the left leg.
   b. Support the client's right side as the client is asked to stand up.
   c. Assess the client's right hip and leg.
   d. Administer pain medication.

   Rationale for your selection: _____
   _____
   _____
   _____

ANSWER KEY FOR
APPLYING CRITICAL THINKING SKILLS TO TEST QUESTIONS

HELPFUL HINTS: Read all test questions carefully. Identify key words in the question that will guide you in answering the question. In these test questions the **key words** to consider are **"most important," "priority initially,"** and **"priority."** Compare your rationale with the one in the test question.

1. The nurse is caring for an 82-year-old client who is 1 day postop left hip replacement. The client has a primary IV infusing at 100 mL/hr, a patient-controlled analgesic device, and a urinary catheter. After assessing the client, the nurse determines that the client is pleasant and cooperative but forgetful. In the afternoon, the nurse notes that the client has become increasingly restless. It is most important for the nurse to
   a. apply a vest restraint.
   b. notify the physician.
   c. check the patient-controlled analgesic device.
   d. assess the client's medical history for dementia.

   Rationale: The answer is (c). Pain may be a contributing factor to the client's restlessness. The patient-controlled analgesic device should be checked to see whether the client has used it to control the pain. Options (a), (b), and (d) are not appropriate interventions.

2. The nurse is delegating the care of a 79-year-old client 2 days postop hip replacement to a nursing assistant who routinely works on a medical unit. Which instruction given to the nursing assistant is of priority initially?
   a. Have the client cough and deep breathe q2h.
   b. Total the intake and output at 1400.
   c. Use a fracture bedpan for toileting needs.
   d. Wash the client's skin with a mild soap.

   Rationale: The answer is (c). A fracture bedpan will minimize putting stress on the hip area and prevent hip dislocation. Options (a), (b), and (d) are important, but instructing a new nursing assistant on how to prevent complications on an unfamiliar unit is of priority.

3. The nurse is assisting a client to get out of a chair after having a right hip replacement 3 days ago. The client suddenly complains of pain and tells the nurse that it hurts too much to walk. Which nursing intervention is of priority?
   a. Encourage the client to put most of the weight on the left leg.
   b. Support the client's right side as the client is asked to stand up.
   c. Assess the client's right hip and leg.
   d. Administer pain medication.

   Rationale: The answer is (c). Increased pain may indicate hip dislocation. Options (a), (b), and (d) are good interventions, but the nurse should assess the surgical site before continuing with any other intervention.

2-22 THE PATIENT WITH A FRACTURED TIBIA

1300 Transfer Handoff Report:

 Mr. W, 26 years old, was admitted with a left fractured tibia. He had surgery and is now being transferred to the orthopedic unit. He has a long leg cast on the left leg. You are assigned to Mr. W as he is taken into his room. He is alert, the left leg cast is damp and clean, and IV of lactated Ringer's is infusing into his right forearm at 125 mL/hr. The PCA is infusing and the IV is patent.

The following patient care plan information is available:

VS q4h I & O (✓) Neurovascular cks (circ. movement, sensation, temp) q2h for 48 hours Elevate left leg on (1) pillow	1 L lactated Ringer's q10h—discontinue when taking fluids well Teach crutch walking in AM by physical therapy	Diet: Clear liquids → Reg. Medications IV pump PCA: Hydromorphone 0.2 mg/hr continuous infusion

Prioritize the following five **recommended nursing interventions** as you would do them to take care of Mr. W. Write a number in the box to identify the order of your interventions (#1 = first intervention, #2 = second intervention, etc.), and state a **rationale** for each intervention.

INTERVENTIONS	PRIORITY #	RATIONALE
• Take VS, assess pain level, pulse ox	☐	_____
• Neurovascular assessment of both extremities	☐	_____
• Assess cast for dryness, signs of drainage, and sharp edges	☐	_____
• Use palms of hands to elevate cast on a pillow	☐	_____
• Teach isometric exercises	☐	_____

KEY POINTS TO CONSIDER _____

_____

_____

_____

On the morning of the first postop day, you note the following:
1. Mr. W states his pain level is 3 out of 10
2. Left pedal pulses present, edema 2+
3. Capillary refill greater than 2 seconds, moves left toes
4. Taking fluids and voiding quantity sufficient
5. MD orders CPK, LDH, and AST

Collaborative Learning Activity: With a partner, **do the following: (1) select** the **one nursing diagnosis** that is a priority at this time, **(2) provide a rationale** for your selection, and **(3) list the nursing interventions** that assist you to meet the needs of the patient.

All of the following nursing diagnoses may apply to Mr. W:

Risk for injury, Deficient knowledge, Risk for infection, Risk for impaired skin integrity, Impaired physical mobility, Fear, Ineffective peripheral tissue perfusion, Acute pain, Activity intolerance, Impaired tissue integrity, Anxiety, Risk for peripheral neurovascular dysfunction

Nursing Diagnosis	Rationale	Nursing Interventions

Mr. W refuses lunch and you assess: complaints of increased pain 8 out of 10, especially with passive elevation of the leg. C/o numbness and tingling, left foot cool, pedal pulse weak

On the basis of this new information, identify and write the **priority problem** in the box below. Then, starting with the small box labeled **#1, prioritize** the **nursing interventions** for this situation and **identify** your follow-up action plan for Mr. W.

NURSING INTERVENTIONS

A. Inform MD stat

B. Prepare to have cast bivalved

C. Ensure that left extremity is at heart level

D. Monitor left pedal pulse

E. Take VS

F. Stay with patient

DECISION-MAKING DIAGRAM

New Action Plan

#1 #2 #3 #4 #5 #6

Priority Problem

NOTES _____

_____

2-23 THE PATIENT WITH CATARACT SURGERY

S	Mrs. G, 72 years old, has senile cataracts and has been instilling mydriatic eye drops. Her vision has progressively worsened and she is scheduled today for a right cataract extraction at the outpatient clinic. The MD orders the following preop preparation: NPO; instill mydriatic and cycloplegic eye drops 1 hour before surgery; diazepam 5 mg po 1 hour before surgery. Mrs. G arrives at the outpatient clinic at 0800, and she is scheduled for surgery at 1000. Mrs. G's daughter will stay with her at home on the day of surgery.
B	Mrs. G is a widow and lives alone. She is an active senior citizen and participates in several volunteer organizations. She has diabetes mellitus type 2 for 30 years and takes glipizide 5 mg po daily.

Prioritize the following five **recommended nursing interventions** as you would do them to take care of Mrs. G. Write a number in the box to identify the order of your interventions (#1 = first intervention, #2 = second intervention, etc.), and state a **rationale** for each intervention.

INTERVENTIONS	PRIORITY #	RATIONALE
• Provide information regarding preop preparation	☐	_____ _____ _____
• Begin to instill ordered eye drops	☐	_____ _____ _____
• Have patient void	☐	_____ _____ _____
• Take VS	☐	_____ _____ _____
⚠ • Ensure that the surgical consent is signed before initiating preop preparation	☐	_____ _____ _____

KEY POINTS TO CONSIDER _____

_____

_____

_____

Mrs. G had an intraocular lens implant and is taken to a room for monitoring. She has an eye patch on her right eye and you assess the following:
1. Pain level 0, P 88, BP 130/82, pulse ox 96%
2. Eye patch clean and dry
3. Readily responds to verbal stimuli

Collaborative Learning Activity: With a partner, **do the following: (1) select the one nursing diagnosis** that is a priority at this time, **(2) provide a rationale** for your selection, and **(3) list the nursing interventions** that assist you to meet the needs of the patient.

All of the following nursing diagnoses may apply to Mrs. G:

Risk for injury, Deficient knowledge, Fear, Anxiety, Risk for infection, Ineffective health maintenance, Impaired home maintenance

Nursing Diagnosis	Rationale	Nursing Interventions

Mrs. G is discharged and given eye drops and eye patches for daily use. Mrs. G and her daughter are given postop instructions. Mrs. G's daughter will take Mrs. G home and stay with her today and will visit every day during the week. On the third postop day, the office nurse calls Mrs G.

Based on the questions asked by the office nurse and Mrs. G's responses, identify the response that requires further follow-up. Provide a rationale for the questions asked by the office nurse.

Office Nurse Follow-Up Questions	Mrs. G's Responses
1. Your eye drops are ordered 4 times per day. Are you able to put them in yourself?	1. I put the morning and afternoon drops in and then my daughter helps with the evening and night eye drops.
2. How often are you taking the medication acetaminophen for pain?	2. I took one tablet last night but have not used any this morning.
3. Are you having any discharge from the eye?	3. I have drainage that is clear and I do have some itching.
4. It is important that you do not pick up heavy objects or bend from the waist.	4. I am taking it easy. The only problem I have is some constipation.

Question 1 Rationale: _____

_____

Question 2 Rationale: _____

_____

Question 3 Rationale: _____

_____

Question 4 Rationale: _____

_____

2-24 THE PATIENT WITH A SEIZURE DISORDER

1600 Transfer Handoff Report:

S	Mr. M, 20 years old, fell at home and lost consciousness. He was just transferred to the neurology unit from the emergency department. He is aware and alert, VS at 1530 are T 97.8°F, P 76, R 20, BP 120/76, pulse ox 98%, pain level 0. The MD orders include seizure precautions, bed rest, soft diet, VS, and neurologic checks q4h. He has a saline lock on the left hand. He is anxious about being admitted.
B	20-year-old male fell at home and was brought to the emergency department after it was noticed that he had lost consciousness for a few seconds. In the emergency department he indicated that he did not remember falling. His family history is significant for seizure disorders. Diagnostic studies included an electroencephalogram, magnetic resonance imaging, serum blood glucose, complete blood cell count, electrolytes, blood urea nitrogen, and urinalysis drug screening.

You begin your assessment by following the recommended nursing interventions.

Prioritize the following five **recommended nursing interventions** as you would do them to initially take care of Mr. M. Write a number in the box to identify the order of your interventions (#1 = first intervention, #2 = second intervention, etc.), and state a **rationale** for each intervention.

INTERVENTIONS	PRIORITY #	RATIONALE
• Orient Mr. M to his room	☐	
• Assess neurologic status	☐	
• Implement seizure precautions	☐	
• Obtain admitting history	☐	
• Inform patient of pertinent MD orders	☐	

KEY POINTS TO CONSIDER _____

_____

_____

_____

Priority Setting and Decision Making — 2

Mr. M is diagnosed with a seizure disorder and is started on divalproex sodium. In speaking with Mr. M you gather the following:

1. Mr. M says that he has had similar episodes but never told anyone.
2. He remembers seeing "spots" before the episode.
3. No one in his family talked much about the relative who had seizures.

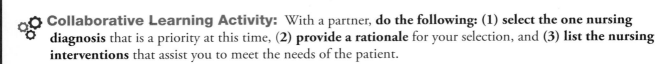 **Collaborative Learning Activity:** With a partner, **do the following: (1) select the one nursing diagnosis** that is a priority at this time, (2) **provide a rationale** for your selection, and (3) **list the nursing interventions** that assist you to meet the needs of the patient.

All of the following nursing diagnoses may apply to Mr. M:

Ineffective coping, Ineffective airway clearance, Risk for injury, Readiness for enhanced knowledge: seizure disorder, Social isolation, Fear, Anxiety, Ineffective health maintenance, Risk for aspiration

Nursing Diagnosis	Rationale	Nursing Interventions

Several hours after admission, you hear a "cry" coming from Mr. M's room. You assess the following as you walk into the room: Tonic-clonic movements of the body, loss of consciousness, excessive salivation, some cyanosis, urinary incontinence, teeth clenched with cessation of tonic-clonic movements after 3 minutes.

On the basis of the situation just described, identify and write the **priority problem** in the box below. Then, starting with the small box labeled **#1, prioritize** the **nursing interventions** for this situation and identify your follow-up action plan for Mr. M.

NURSING INTERVENTIONS   **DECISION-MAKING DIAGRAM**

A. Maintain a quiet environment

B. Assess for injury

C. Check airway patency   **New Action Plan**

                                        #1   #2   #3   #4   #5   #6
D. Record findings

E. Turn to side

F. Reorient patient   **NOTES** _____

Priority Problem   _____

APPLYING CRITICAL THINKING SKILLS TO TEST QUESTIONS

INSTRUCTIONS: Circle the one best answer for each test question. Write your rationale for selecting the answer. To enhance your learning and test-taking skills, discuss your answer and rationale with a partner. The answer and the rationale can be found on the back of this page.

2 Priority Setting and Decision Making

1. The nurse documents the following after observing a client have a tonic-clonic seizure: "0930 Found client having jerky, involuntary movements of upper and lower extremities lasting 2 minutes, frothy saliva oozing from mouth, incontinent of urine." Which statement best describes the nurse's documentation? The documentation
   a. is appropriate and describes the observations seen.
   b. should include the client's response and nursing interventions.
   c. should just indicate that the client had a tonic-clonic seizure.
   d. is lacking whether the client had an aura experience before the seizure.

   Rationale for your selection: _____
   _____
   _____
   _____

2. The nurse admits a client who is having uncontrolled generalized tonic-clonic seizures. In planning for potential complications, which nursing intervention is of priority?
   a. Place bed in low position.
   b. Have suction equipment available.
   c. Maintain side rails up at all times.
   d. Maintain a quiet environment.

   Rationale for your selection: _____
   _____
   _____
   _____

3. The nurse is caring for a client who is on phenytoin (Dilantin) 200 mg po tid and phenobarbital 20 mg po tid. Which assessment finding is most indicative of a common side effect of these medications?
   a. Gums red and swollen
   b. Complaints of constipation
   c. Respiratory depression
   d. Skin rash

   Rationale for your selection: _____
   _____
   _____
   _____

2 Priority Setting and Decision Making

ANSWER KEY FOR APPLYING CRITICAL THINKING SKILLS TO TEST QUESTIONS

HELPFUL HINTS: Read all test questions carefully. Identify key words in the question that will guide you in answering the question. In these test questions the **key words** to consider are **"best," "priority,"** and **"most indicative."** Compare your rationale with the one in the test question.

1. The nurse documents the following after observing a client have a tonic-clonic seizure: "0930 Found client having jerky, involuntary movements of upper and lower extremities lasting 2 minutes, frothy saliva oozing from mouth, incontinent of urine." Which statement best describes the nurse's documentation? The documentation
   a. is appropriate and describes the observations seen.
   b. should include the client's response and nursing interventions.
   c. should just indicate that the client had a tonic-clonic seizure.
   d. is lacking whether the client had an aura experience before the seizure.

   Rationale: The answer is (b). Documentation should include what is observed, the nursing interventions, and the client's response/reaction. Options (a), (c), and (d) do not include all the components necessary for legal documentation.

2. The nurse admits a client who is having uncontrolled generalized tonic-clonic seizures. In planning for potential complications, which nursing intervention is of priority?
   a. Place bed in low position.
   b. Have suction equipment available.
   c. Maintain side rails up at all times.
   d. Maintain a quiet environment.

   Rationale: The answer is (b). Suction equipment is necessary to clear oral secretions after the seizure and prevent aspiration. Options (a), (c), and (d) are important, but preventing aspiration is of priority.

3. The nurse is caring for a client who is on phenytoin (Dilantin) 200 mg po tid and phenobarbital 20 mg po tid. Which assessment finding is most indicative of a common side effect of these medications?
   a. Gums red and swollen
   b. Complaints of constipation
   c. Respiratory depression
   d. Skin rash

   Rationale: The answer is (a). Gingival hyperplasia is a common side effect seen with the administration of phenytoin. Meticulous oral hygiene is an important intervention. Option (b) is not a common side effect. Option (c) is a toxic reaction to phenobarbital, and option (d) is a toxic reaction to phenytoin.

2-25 THE PATIENT WITH A DO-NOT-RESUSCITATE ORDER

0700 Handoff Report:

> **S** Mr. B, 83 years old, has terminal esophageal cancer. His current respirations are 10 and he last received IV morphine sulfate at 6:00 AM. PEG residual was 125 mL and the tube feeding was stopped at 0600. The IV has 200 mL left.

The following patient care plan information is available:

Activity: Bed rest Vital signs: q4h I & O q8h Oral suction prn Lives with son Hospital Day: #4	IV: 0.9% NS q12h Urinary catheter inserted on admission Code status: DNR	PEG tube insertion: 3 days ago 1/2 strength formula at 50 mL/hr Ck residual q4h, if greater than 100 mL, hold feeding for 1 hour PRN medications: Morphine sulfate 2 mg direct IV injection q2h prn pain

Prioritize the following five **recommended nursing interventions** as you would do them to initially take care of Mr. B. Write a number in the box to identify the order of your interventions (#1 = first intervention, #2 = second intervention, etc.), and state a **rationale** for each intervention.

INTERVENTIONS	PRIORITY #	RATIONALE
• Assess PEG tube residual	☐	_____
• Take VS and pain level	☐	_____
• Assess IV site and IV fluid level	☐	_____
• Perform a body system assessment	☐	_____
• Assess patency of urinary catheter and output	☐	_____

KEY POINTS TO CONSIDER _____

_____

_____

_____

2 Priority Setting and Decision Making

At 11:00 AM Mr. B manifested the following signs and symptoms:
1. VS: P 76, R14, BP 118/64, pulse ox 93%, pain level difficult to assess
2. Responds appropriately but is weak and lethargic, no grimacing
3. Urine is dark yellow; output 125 mL since 7:00 AM
4. Shortness of breath when turning; irregular breathing pattern

Collaborative Learning Activity: With a partner, **do the following: (1) select the one nursing diagnosis** that is a priority at this time, **(2) provide a rationale** for your selection, and **(3) list the nursing interventions** that assist you to meet the needs of the patient.

All of the following nursing diagnoses may apply to Mr. B:

Risk for infection, Acute pain, Anxiety, Impaired gas exchange, Imbalanced nutrition: less than body requirements, Risk for deficient fluid volume, Risk for impaired skin integrity, Ineffective peripheral tissue perfusion, Activity intolerance, Powerlessness, Social isolation

Nursing Diagnosis	Rationale	Nursing Interventions

At **2:00 PM** Mr. B is unresponsive to verbal stimuli. You assessed: VS: P 36, R 9, BP 80/50, pulse ox 86%. Urine output unchanged since 11:00 AM. Lower extremities cool with cyanosis.

Based on the **2:00 PM** assessment, identify and write the **priority problem** in the box below. Then, starting with the small box labeled **#1, prioritize** the **nursing interventions** for this situation and **identify** your plan for follow-up care for Mr. B.

NURSING INTERVENTIONS

A. Monitor VS

B. Check NCP for religious/cultural requests

C. Report findings to physician

D. Notify relatives

E. Provide comfort measures

F. Record findings

DECISION-MAKING DIAGRAM

New Action Plan

#1   #2   #3   #4   #5   #6

Priority Problem

NOTES _____

2-26 LEGAL CONSIDERATIONS

1500 Handoff Report:

S	Mrs. L is one day postop total abdominal hysterectomy. Morphine sulfate 5 mg is ordered direct IV injection q3h prn pain since the PCA has been discontinued. She is on a soft diet and has not voided since the urinary catheter was removed at noon. Her last pain shot was administered at 2:00 PM. She ambulates with assistance. VS at noon are T 99°F, P 82, R 22, BP 130/76, pulse ox 96%. The incentive spirometer is at the bedside.
B	A healthy 42-year-old female is admitted for total abdominal hysterectomy. She has been having heavy menstrual flow and irregular periods. GYN examination reveals uterine fibroids. She has a family history of uterine and cervical cancer.
A	The abdominal dressing is stained with dried dark red drainage. Fine crackles are audible in the lower bases of the lung fields. She states her pain level is 4 out of 10 at 1600.
R	The following nursing interventions are recommended:

Prioritize the following five **recommended nursing interventions** as you, the nurse, would do them to initially take care of Mrs. L. Write a number in the box to identify the order of your interventions (#1 = first intervention, #2 = second intervention, etc.), and state a **rationale** for each intervention.

INTERVENTIONS	PRIORITY #	RATIONALE
• Inform Mrs. L to drink a minimum of four 8-ounce glasses of water for the shift	☐	_____
• Cough and deep breathe; demonstrate abdominal splinting; use incentive spirometer q1h	☐	_____
• Ambulate to the bathroom	☐	_____
• Take VS	☐	_____
• Assess abdomen and surgical dressing	☐	_____

KEY POINTS TO CONSIDER _____

Mrs. L voids 400 mL after ambulating to the bathroom and states that she feels much better. She relates the following to you:

1. Her mother had a hysterectomy but died 10 days after from surgical complications.
2. She is glad that she does not have to worry about irregular periods any more.
3. She fully trusts her doctor but wonders whether the right thing was done.
4. She lives alone.

Collaborative Learning Activity: With a partner, **do the following: (1) select the one nursing diagnosis** that is a priority at this time, **(2) provide a rationale** for your selection, and **(3) list the nursing interventions** that assist you to meet the needs of the patient.

All of the following nursing diagnoses may apply to Mrs. L:

> Risk for infection, Acute pain, Anxiety, Ineffective breathing pattern, Imbalanced nutrition: less than body requirements, Disturbed body image, Sexual dysfunction, Impaired skin integrity, Risk for activity intolerance, Deficient knowledge

Nursing Diagnosis	Rationale	Nursing Interventions

At 6:00 PM Mrs. L states that she is having pain. Mrs. L's pain is at a level of 8 out of 10. She has not received any pain medication since 2:00 PM. You take out an ampule labeled hydromorphone 10 mg/mL and administer 0.5 mL to Mrs. L. After the administration of the hydromorphone you realize that hydromorphone is not morphine sulfate.

Based on the situation just described, identify and write the **priority problem** in the box below. Then, starting with the small box labeled **#1, prioritize** the **nursing interventions** for this situation and **identify** your follow-up action plan for Mrs. L.

NURSING INTERVENTIONS

⚠ A. Stay with the patient

B. Record drug and amount given

C. Monitor respiratory depression and circulatory collapse

D. Follow agency policy for reporting error

E. Notify your RN and instructor stat

F. Notify physician stat

DECISION-MAKING DIAGRAM

New Action Plan

#1 #2 #3 #4 #5 #6

Priority Problem

NOTES _____

SECTION 3

Critical Thinking Model Application

3-1 PATIENT WITH SMALL BOWEL RESECTION

0700 Handoff Report:

S	Mr. A, a 72-year-old male, is 2 days postop small bowel resection. His NG tube is connected to continuous low wall suction and has drained 75 mL of tan-colored fluid. Vital signs at 0600: T 99.6° F, P 90, R 28, BP 160/94, pulse ox 94%. He has D5/0.45 NS with 20 mEq KCl infusing at 125 mL in the right forearm, 300 mL are left. He is using the PCA with relief, pain level 2.
B	History and physical indicate that Mr. A suffered from Crohn's disease, experiencing watery bloody diarrhea.
A	Abd soft, faint bowel sounds present ×2 quadrants. He slept most of the night and is now sitting in a chair. SOB was noted when he was transferred to the chair. Lung sounds diminished in the right lower lung.

The following information is obtained from Mr. A's electronic medical record:

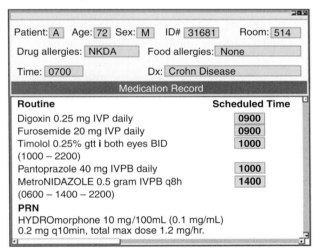

Patient: A Age: 72 Sex: M ID# 31681 Room: 514

Drug allergies: NKDA Food allergies: None

Time: 0700 Dx: Crohn Disease

Medication Record

Routine	Scheduled Time
Digoxin 0.25 mg IVP daily	0900
Furosemide 20 mg IVP daily	0900
Timolol 0.25% gtt **i** both eyes BID (1000 – 2200)	1000
Pantoprazole 40 mg IVPB daily	1000
MetroNIDAZOLE 0.5 gram IVPB q8h (0600 – 1400 – 2200)	1400
PRN	
HYDROmorphone 10 mg/100mL (0.1 mg/mL) 0.2 mg q10min, total max dose 1.2 mg/hr.	

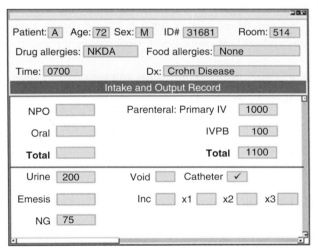

Patient: A Age: 72 Sex: M ID# 31681 Room: 514

Drug allergies: NKDA Food allergies: None

Time: 0700 Dx: Crohn Disease

Intake and Output Record

NPO		Parenteral: Primary IV	1000
Oral		IVPB	100
Total		**Total**	1100

Urine	200	Void		Catheter	✓
Emesis		Inc		x1	x2	x3
NG	75				

⚙ Collaborative Learning Activity: With a partner, **use the clinical situation and the electronic medical record** to:

1. Identify the pertinent patient information made known to you in the handoff *report*. →	2. Identify the pertinent patient information made known to you from the *electronic medical record*. →	3. Review the data in columns 1 and 2 and identify information that needs follow-up.

It is 0730 when the handoff report is completed. **Prioritize** your plan of care for the morning:

Time	Plan of Care

1200 nursing assessment: Oriented ×3, skin WNL, capillary refill less than 3 sec, turgor good, mucous membranes moist, pinkish, T 99°F, P 88 and slightly irregular, R 20, BP 164/94, pulse ox 96%. NG draining brownish fluid 100 mL since 0800. Bowel sounds present ×4, abd soft. Foley catheter draining clear yellow urine.

Mr. A has minimal complaints and is visited by the physician at 1200. The physician writes the following orders:

Remove Foley now
Enc. incentive spirometer q1h ×10
Discontinue NG tube
Discontinue furosemide
Discontinue IV digoxin, start digoxin 0.25 mg po daily
Hgb & Hct today
Clear liquid diet

IP **1. Identify the nursing interventions that require immediate follow-up.**	**2. Identify the nursing actions that you can delegate/assign to unlicensed personnel.**

Critical Reflection: To promote **safe nursing practice**, the handoff report at 0700 and the electronic medical record:

☐ communicated sufficient information to provide continuous care to the patient.

☐ lacked the following: _____

_____

_____

3-2 PATIENT WITH GI BLEED AND ETOH ABUSE

0700 Handoff Report:

S	The patient is 43 years old and was admitted yesterday from the ED after experiencing GI bleeding. He is NPO and has an NG tube connected to continuous low wall suction. The NG tube drained 100 mL of dark reddish drainage.
B	Patient has a long history of ETOH abuse. He had been drinking the day of admission.
A	Vital signs at 6:00 AM are T 97.4° F, P 96, R 18, BP 130/86, pulse ox 96%. Pain level 0. A unit of whole blood is infusing and should be finished by 9:00 AM. His current Hgb is 8.6, and he is more restless this morning.

The following information is obtained from the patient's electronic medical record:

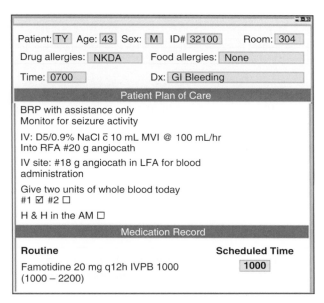

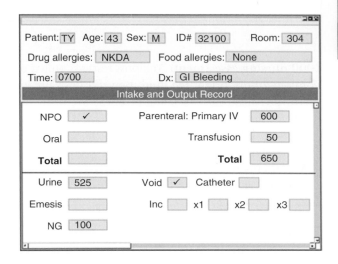

⚙ **Collaborative Learning Activity:** With a partner, **use the clinical situation and the electronic medical record** to:

1. Identify the pertinent patient information made known to you in the handoff *report*. →	2. Identify the pertinent patient information made known to you from the *electronic medical record*. →	3. Review the data in columns 1 and 2 and identify information that needs follow-up.

It is 0730 when the handoff report is completed. **Prioritize** your plan of care for the morning:

Time	Plan of Care

1000 nursing assessment: Anxious, restless, pulled out NG tube. Physician called. VS: P 100, R 26, BP 146/90. Vomited 20 mL bright red fluid. Bowel sounds present ×4, abd soft. Transfusion #2 infusing at 25 gtt/min.

The physician calls back and gives the following orders:

Oxygen at 2 L/min/NP

Reinsert NG tube

ABG, serum electrolytes Mg^{++}, BG, serum ammonia level, BUN

VS and neuro checks q2h

Chlordiazepoxide HCl 50 mg IV push stat

IP 1. Identify the nursing interventions that require immediate follow-up.	2. Identify the nursing actions that you can delegate/assign to unlicensed personnel.

Critical Reflection: To implement safe nursing interventions, identify the signs and symptoms associated with alcohol withdrawal syndrome as absence of alcohol progresses.

First 12 hrs: _____

12–24 hrs: _____

12–48 hrs: _____

48 hrs or more: _____

3-3 PATIENT WITH DEHYDRATION, FEVER, DO-NOT-RESUSCITATE ORDER

3 Critical Thinking Model Application

1600 Handoff Report:

S	The patient was admitted today for dehydration. She is 88 years old and has a stage IV pressure ulcer on her sacrum. The hydrocolloid dressing was applied today. A 2 cm × 2 cm eschar is on her left heel. She weighs 90 lbs and she refused her lunch. An IV was started at 1400. You have 750 mL left. She is a sweet little lady, quiet, and at times forgetful. Her admission lab results just came in, her Hgb is 9.6, Hct 27, WBC 11,000, and K⁺ 4.5. Her physician is coming later this evening.
B	Patient has been living alone. Family reports that they have noticed a significant mental decline for the last 3 months. Daughter brought patient to the emergency room this morning.

The following information is obtained from the patient's electronic medical record:

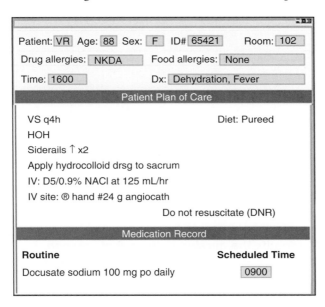

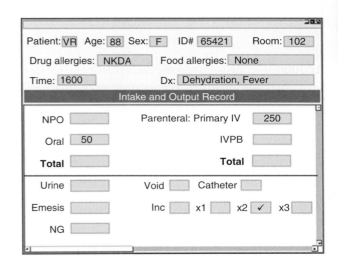

⚙ **Collaborative Learning Activity:** With a partner, **use the clinical situation and the electronic medical record** to:

1. Identify the pertinent patient information made known to you in the handoff *report*.	2. Identify the pertinent patient information made known to you from the *electronic medical record*.	3. Review the data in columns 1 and 2 and identify information that needs follow-up.

It is 1630 when the handoff report is completed. **Prioritize** your plan of care for the next 4 hours:

Time	Plan of Care

At 2000 the nursing assistant reports that the patient is restless and trying to get out of bed. You document the following assessment: Speech incoherent, skin warm, flushed. VS: T 101°F, P 92, R 24, BP 108/60, pulse ox 88%. Incontinent of dark-colored urine with strong odor. Physician called. The following orders are given:

VS q2h, I & O
Acetaminophen 325 mg po q4h prn temperature greater than 100.4°F
Enc. fluid intake
Ceftriaxone 1 g IVPB qAM

IP

1. Identify the nursing interventions that require immediate follow-up.	2. Identify the nursing actions that you can delegate/assign to unlicensed personnel.

Critical Reflection: To promote patient-centered care, list nursing interventions that you could independently implement for this patient:

_____

_____

_____

3-4 PATIENT WITH FRACTURED TIBIA AND ASTHMA

2300 Handoff Report:

 S The patient in 205 was admitted with a fractured right tibia and is 1 day postop. He has a cast on. He has been quiet most of the evening. He just started coughing and is experiencing some SOB. He says he has a history of asthma and that he gets this way every now and then. I did not detect any wheezing. Vital signs are T 98.8°F, P 90, R 28, BP 140/88, pulse ox 92%, pain level 3 out of 10 on the pain scale. Circulation, movement, and sensation are WNL in the right leg.

The following information is obtained from the patient's electronic medical record:

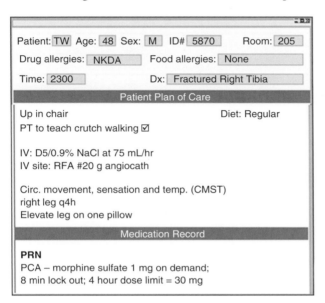

Patient: TW Age: 48 Sex: M ID# 5870 Room: 205

Drug allergies: NKDA Food allergies: None

Time: 2300 Dx: Fractured Right Tibia

Patient Plan of Care

Up in chair Diet: Regular
PT to teach crutch walking ☑

IV: D5/0.9% NaCl at 75 mL/hr
IV site: RFA #20 g angiocath

Circ. movement, sensation and temp. (CMST)
right leg q4h
Elevate leg on one pillow

Medication Record

PRN
PCA – morphine sulfate 1 mg on demand;
8 min lock out; 4 hour dose limit = 30 mg

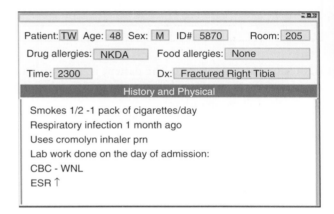

Patient: TW Age: 48 Sex: M ID# 5870 Room: 205

Drug allergies: NKDA Food allergies: None

Time: 2300 Dx: Fractured Right Tibia

History and Physical

Smokes 1/2 -1 pack of cigarettes/day
Respiratory infection 1 month ago
Uses cromolyn inhaler prn
Lab work done on the day of admission:
CBC - WNL
ESR ↑

Collaborative Learning Activity: With a partner, **use the clinical situation and the electronic medical record** to:

1. Identify the pertinent patient information made known to you in the handoff *report*.	2. Identify the pertinent patient information made known to you from the *electronic medical record.*	3. Review the data in columns 1 and 2 and identify information that needs follow-up.

It is 2330 as you leave the report room. **Prioritize** your plan of care for the next 3 hours:

Time	Plan of Care

0200 nursing assessment: The patient is beginning to cough more frequently and complains of chest tightness. Respiratory assessment indicates inspiratory and expiratory wheezes in bilateral lungs. You call the physician and obtain the following orders:

    IV D5/0.9% NaCl at 125 mL/hr
    Oxygen at 2 L/min/NP
    Albuterol inhaler 2 puffs q4h
    Metaproterenol nebulizer treatment 0.3 mL (5%) in 2.5 mL NS q4h prn
    ABG, sputum for eosinophils
    Methylprednisolone sodium 125 mg IVP q6h
    Check oxygen saturation with pulse oximeter q2h
    Call physician with ABG results

1. Identify the nursing interventions that require immediate follow-up.	2. ☑ Identify the nursing actions that you can delegate/assign to unlicensed personnel.

Critical Reflection: To promote patient-centered care, list nursing interventions that you could independently implement for this patient:

3-5 PATIENT WITH PANCREATITIS AND CENTRAL LINE

1500 Handoff Report:

 S Mrs. C, 42 years old, was admitted earlier today with the diagnosis of acute pancreatitis. She had mid-epigastric pain with nausea and vomiting on admission. Her latest vital signs are T 38°C, P 108, R 26, BP 110/60, pulse ox 97%. Bowel sounds are hypoactive. I gave her HYDROmorphone 2 mg at 2:00 PM. A central line was inserted; you have 800 mL left in the IV of lactated Ringer's The NG is draining brownish fluid.

The following information is obtained from Mrs C's electronic medical record:

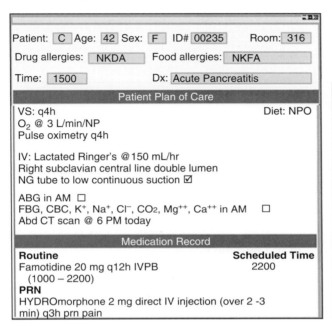

Patient: C Age: 42 Sex: F ID# 00235   Room: 316

Drug allergies: NKDA   Food allergies: NKFA

Time: 1500   Dx: Acute Pancreatitis

Patient Plan of Care

VS: q4h   Diet: NPO
O_2 @ 3 L/min/NP
Pulse oximetry q4h

IV: Lactated Ringer's @150 mL/hr
Right subclavian central line double lumen
NG tube to low continuous suction ☑

ABG in AM ☐
FBG, CBC, K^+, Na^+, Cl^-, CO_2, Mg^{++}, Ca^{++} in AM   ☐
Abd CT scan @ 6 PM today

Medication Record

Routine	Scheduled Time
Famotidine 20 mg q12h IVPB (1000 – 2200)	2200

PRN
HYDROmorphone 2 mg direct IV injection (over 2 -3 min) q3h prn pain

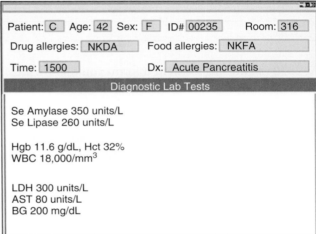

Patient: C Age: 42 Sex: F ID# 00235   Room: 316

Drug allergies: NKDA   Food allergies: NKFA

Time: 1500   Dx: Acute Pancreatitis

Diagnostic Lab Tests

Se Amylase 350 units/L
Se Lipase 260 units/L

Hgb 11.6 g/dL, Hct 32%
WBC 18,000/mm^3

LDH 300 units/L
AST 80 units/L
BG 200 mg/dL

3 Critical Thinking Model Application

Collaborative Learning Activity: With a partner, **use the clinical situation and the electronic medical record** to:

1. Identify the pertinent patient information made known to you in the handoff *report.*	2. Identify the pertinent patient information made known to you from the *electronic medical record.*	3. Review the data in columns 1 and 2 and identify information that needs follow-up.

It is 1600. Prioritize your plan of care for the next 3 hours:

Time	Plan of Care

At 2030 the nursing assistant informs you that Mrs. C is complaining of pain and is restless. You note that she has not had a pain shot in the last 3 hours. You walk into the room to assess her and to give her the pain medication injection. She turns over quickly and pulls out the central line.

IP	1. Identify the nursing interventions that you would implement immediately at the bedside.	2. Identify the follow-up nursing actions. Document the incident that should be included in the nursing notes.
Nurse's Notes		

Critical Reflection: Mrs. C is very anxious after the central line was pulled and asks you if she needs to have that "central line" inserted again. To provide patient-centered care at this time, list two questions that would support Mrs. C's current needs.

1. _____

_____

_____

2. _____

_____

_____

_____

3-6 PATIENT WITH A HEAD TRAUMA

0800 Handoff Report:

S	The patient is a young man who was transferred from the ICU yesterday. He was in a motor vehicle accident (MVA) 14 days ago. He had some head trauma and subsequent evacuation of a subdural hematoma.
A	He is unconscious, unresponsive to painful stimuli, and has flaccid extremities. Pupils round, sluggish reaction to light. He has several abrasions on his face and several bruised areas on his shoulders and chest from the accident. Vital signs are T 97.8°F, P 94, R 24, BP 124/80, pulse ox 94%. Mother at bedside; she questions everything you do.

The following information is obtained from the patient's electronic medical record:

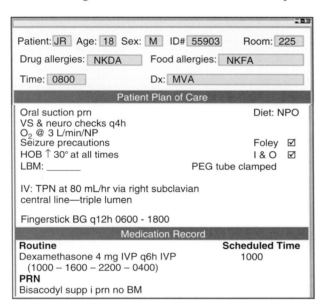

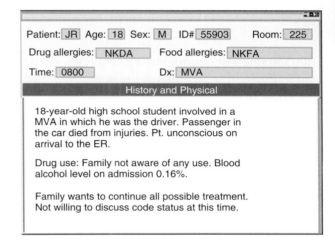

3 Critical Thinking Model Application

⚙ **Collaborative Learning Activity:** With a partner, **use the clinical situation and the electronic medical record** to:

1. Identify the pertinent patient information made known to you in the handoff *report*.	2. Identify the pertinent patient information made known to you from the *electronic medical record.*	3. Review the data in columns 1 and 2 and identify information that needs follow-up.

It is 0830 when the handoff report is completed. **Prioritize** your plan of care for the next 3 hours:

Time	Plan of Care

1400 nursing assessment: Pupil round R ● L ● nonreactive to light. R 12 Cheyne-Stokes, P 80, BP 150/80. Skin warm, jerky movements of the upper extremity noted. The physician writes the following orders:

Oxygen at 12 L/min per non-rebreather mask
Check oxygen saturation q1h
Vital signs q1h
CT scan of the head stat
ABGs stat

IP	1. Identify the nursing interventions that require immediate follow-up.	2. Identify the nursing actions that you can delegate/assign to unlicensed personnel.

Critical Reflection: To provide patient-centered care, list how you would support the mother at this time.

_____

_____

_____

_____

3-7 SENSITIVE POSTMORTEM CARE

0800 Handoff Report:

S	The patient is 52 years old and has bone cancer. She has been requesting pain medication every 2 hours. I gave her morphine sulfate 2 mg this morning at 0630. Her respirations have gone down to 10 during the night. She does not want to be turned. A urinary catheter was inserted in the evening shift. A family member spent the night with her. Latest vital signs at 6:00 AM are T 97°F, P 66, R 12, BP 128/60.
B	Patient's advance directive contains request for DNR.

The following information is obtained from the patient's electronic medical record:

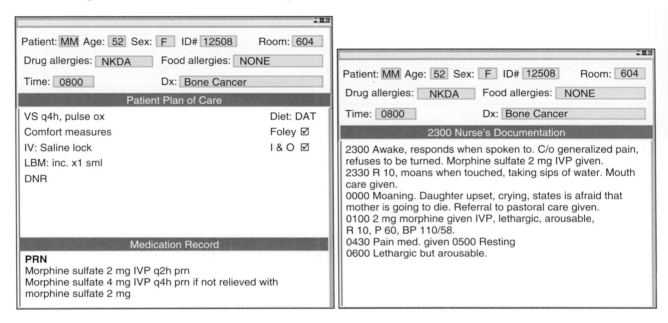

Collaborative Learning Activity: With a partner, **use the clinical situation and the electronic medical record** to:

1. Identify the pertinent patient information made known to you in the handoff *report*.	2. Identify the pertinent patient information made known to you from the *electronic medical record.*	3. Review the data in columns 1 and 2 and identify information that needs follow-up.

It is 0830 when the handoff report is completed. **Prioritize** your plan of care for the next 3 hours:

Time	Plan of Care

At 1230 you return from lunch to learn that the nursing assistant was unable to obtain a pulse on the patient. You assess the following: Unresponsive, skin cool, legs pale with mottling. Pulse not palpable, no apical or BP audible. Family with patient. Physician contacted and pronounced patient dead. Family is making arrangements for a mortuary to pick up the patient within the hour.

1. Identify the nursing interventions that require immediate follow-up.	2. Identify the nursing actions that you can delegate/assign to unlicensed personnel.

Critical Reflection: To provide patient-centered care, identify nursing interventions that support the family during this time.

_____

_____

_____

_____

3-8 PATIENT FALLING WITH COMPLICATIONS

0700 Handoff Report:

 Mrs. F, 79 years old, was in a motor vehicle accident (MVA) 2 days ago. She fractured her right arm. Her right arm is in a cast; circulation, movement, and sensation are fine. She is scheduled to go home this morning. She slept fine and was given HYDROcodone/acetaminophen 5-325 for pain at 0430 AM with relief. VS are WNL and pain level is 1–2 at 6:00 AM.

At 0730 as you complete the handoff reports on your assigned patients, the night nurse tells you that Mrs. F got up to go to the bathroom and fell coming back to bed. She has a slight nosebleed and was given an icepack and assisted back to bed. The physician was called and informed of her falling. He said he would be in later to see her before discharge.

The following information is obtained from Mrs. F's electronic medical record:

3 Critical Thinking
Model Application

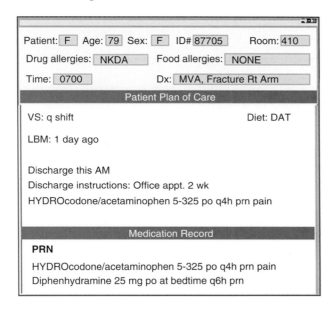

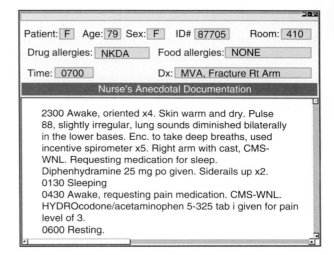

Patient: F   Age: 79   Sex: F   ID# 87705   Room: 410

Drug allergies: NKDA   Food allergies: NONE

Time: 0700   Dx: MVA, Fracture Rt Arm

Patient Plan of Care

VS: q shift   Diet: DAT

LBM: 1 day ago

Discharge this AM
Discharge instructions: Office appt. 2 wk
HYDROcodone/acetaminophen 5-325 po q4h prn pain

Medication Record

PRN

HYDROcodone/acetaminophen 5-325 po q4h prn pain
Diphenhydramine 25 mg po at bedtime q6h prn

Patient: F   Age: 79   Sex: F   ID# 87705   Room: 410

Drug allergies: NKDA   Food allergies: NONE

Time: 0700   Dx: MVA, Fracture Rt Arm

Nurse's Anecdotal Documentation

2300 Awake, oriented x4. Skin warm and dry. Pulse 88, slightly irregular, lung sounds diminished bilaterally in the lower bases. Enc. to take deep breaths, used incentive spirometer x5. Right arm with cast, CMS-WNL. Requesting medication for sleep. Diphenhydramine 25 mg po given. Siderails up x2.
0130 Sleeping
0430 Awake, requesting pain medication. CMS-WNL. HYDROcodone/acetaminophen 5-325 tab i given for pain level of 3.
0600 Resting.

Collaborative Learning Activity: With a partner, **use the clinical situation and the electronic medical record** to:

1. Identify the pertinent patient information made known to you in the handoff *report*.	2. Identify the pertinent patient information made known to you from the *electronic medical record.*	3. Review the data in columns 1 and 2 and identify information that needs follow-up.

It is 0730. Prioritize your plan of care for the next hour:

Time	Plan of Care

At 0830 you note that Mrs. F is lethargic and very slow to respond to verbal stimuli. Skin is cool with slight cyanosis noted on nail beds. P 110 and irregular, R 14 shallow, pulse ox 92%, BP 90/70, which is lower than her usual of 130/88.

IP 1. Identify the nursing interventions that you would plan to implement immediately.	2. Identify the nursing actions that you can delegate/assign to unlicensed personnel.

Critical Reflection: To promote safe nursing practice, the patient report at 0730:

☐ communicated sufficient information regarding the patient's fall and follow-up nursing interventions.

☐ lacked the following: _____

_____

_____

3-9 PATIENT WITH HYPERTENSION AND MEDICATION ERROR

0700 Handoff Report on your assigned patients:

S	Mrs. A is 67 years old and has diabetes mellitus type 1 and hypertension. She is in for a pressure ulcer on her right heel. There is a hydrocolloid dressing that is due to be changed at 1000. VS are stable and her latest BP is 170/108, denies pain, pulse ox 97%. She is on bed rest with the right leg elevated and she only has BRP.
S	Mrs. C is 73 years old and was admitted with dehydration 3 days ago. She is eating and voiding well. There is a possibility that she is going home today. I removed her saline lock; there was some redness at the IV site. She is not on any IV meds, so I decided not to restart. She says that she is going home this afternoon, although there is no order. Her morning vital signs are: T 97°F, P 82, R 18, BP 130/90, pulse ox 98%, pain level 0.

Mrs. A's and Mrs. C's **electronic medication records** contain the following information:

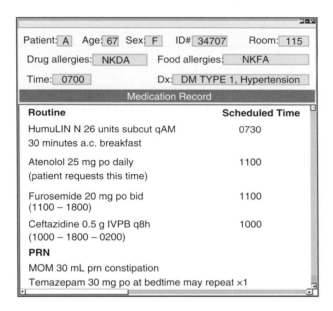

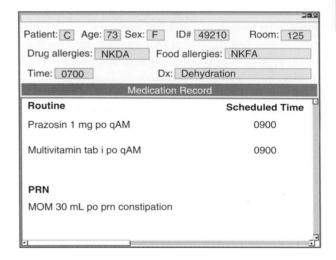

Collaborative Learning Activity: With a partner, **use the clinical situation and the electronic medical record** to:

1. Identify the pertinent patient information made known to you in the handoff *report.*	2. Identify the pertinent patient information made known to you from the *electronic medical record.*	3. Review the data in columns 1 and 2 and identify information that needs follow-up.
Mrs. A: Mrs. C:	Mrs. A: Mrs. C:	Mrs. A: Mrs. C:

3 Critical Thinking Model Application

It is 0800. Prioritize your plan of care for both patients for the next 3 hours:

Time	Plan of Care

You return from lunch at 1200 and Mrs. A is asking for her antihypertensive medication. You know you gave the medication, but she insists that you did not give her the medication. As you investigate, the nursing assistant tells you that Mrs. C is very lethargic and unresponsive. You suddenly realize that you gave Mrs. A's 1100 medications to Mrs. C.

IP	1. Identify the nursing interventions that you would plan to implement immediately.	2. Make a nurse's note entry as to how you might document this incident in the patient's electronic medical record.

Critical Reflection: To promote safe nursing practice in medication administration when caring for multiple patients, identify nursing actions:

_____

_____

_____

3-10 ELDERLY PATIENT WITH MRSA

2300 Handoff Report:

S Mrs. J, 88 years old, was admitted this evening from a skilled nursing facility. The family says the patient was lethargic and confused during their visit. Her admitting vital signs were T 101°F, P 92 and irregular, R 28 and short and shallow, BP 110/70, pulse ox 94%. Unable to accurately assess pain level. Her physician was called for admitting orders and was informed of the UA report from the skilled nursing facility. He will come in tomorrow morning to see her. She was given acetaminophen at 2030 and her current temperature is 100.6°F; she is still slightly confused. She has an IV infusing. She is in a private room.

The following information is obtained from Mrs. J's electronic medical record:

Patient: J Age: 88 Sex: F ID# 00781 Room: 204
Drug allergies: NKDA Food allergies: None
Time: 2300 Dx: UTI, MRSA

Patient Plan of Care

VS q4h Diet: DAT

LBM: On admission

IV: 0.9% NaCl at 75 mL/hr
#24 angiocath RFA

Lab: CBC, chem panel, UA done on admission

Medication Record

PRN
Acetaminophen 325 mg tabs ii po q4h prn temp greater than 101°F

Document from Skilled Nursing Facility

Documentation of latest nurse's notes:

1600 Turned, incontinent of urine, strong urine odor, incontinence pad applied. ———————— *A. Cann LVN*
1700 Family in to visit. Upset, called physician. ———————— *A. Cann LVN*
1830 Transferred to hospital per order. Recent UA culture reports show + MRSA. Unable to contact physician to inform. Copy of report included with transfer. ———*T. Gage RN*

Collaborative Learning Activity: With a partner, **use the clinical situation and the electronic medical record** to:

1. Identify the pertinent patient information made known to you in the handoff *report*.	2. Identify the pertinent patient information made known to you from the *electronic medical record.*	3. Review the data in columns 1 and 2 and identify information that needs follow-up.

3 Critical Thinking Model Application

It is 2330. Prioritize your plan of care for the next hour:

Time	Plan of Care

Mrs. J slept 1 to 2 hours at a time during the night and remains confused. She has developed a productive cough and is expectorating a small amount of thick, creamy, yellow-colored phlegm. Her morning vital signs are T 100.8°F, P 110, R 32, BP 114/82, pulse ox 92%. At 0630 the physician visits and writes the following orders:

Vancomycin 1 gram q12h IVPB
Insert indwelling urinary catheter
Bed rest
Chest x-ray/ECG
Oxygen 2 L/min/NP, pulse oximeter continuous monitoring
I & O, enc. fluid intake

IP **1. Identify the nursing interventions that you would plan to implement immediately.**	**2. Identify the instructions you would give to staff and family in caring for Mrs. J.**

Critical Reflection: To provide patient-centered care, identify nursing interventions that support the patient and family during this time:

_____

_____

_____

_____

_____

3-11 PATIENT WITH VIRAL HEPATITIS

2300 Handoff Report:

> **S** The patient is 27 years old and was admitted this evening. He has been diagnosed with viral hepatitis. He is very jaundiced and his urine is very dark yellow. Intake for the shift was 100 mL and output 300 mL. He does not want to eat. He says he has not had an appetite for several days. The IV was started at 1700 and is on time. His 2000 vital signs are T 37.5°C, P 88, R 24, BP 130/70, pain level 1, pulse ox 98%. He is currently complaining of itching and nausea and I have not medicated him. Lab reports are in the EMR.

The following information is obtained from the patient's electronic medical record:

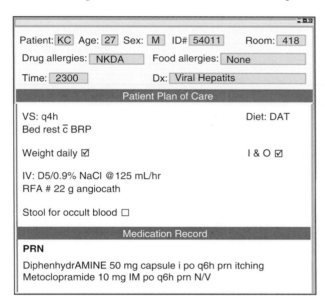

Patient: KC Age: 27 Sex: M ID# 54011 Room: 418
Drug allergies: NKDA Food allergies: None
Time: 2300 Dx: Viral Hepatits

Patient Plan of Care

VS: q4h   Diet: DAT
Bed rest c̄ BRP

Weight daily ☑   I & O ☑

IV: D5/0.9% NaCl @125 mL/hr
RFA # 22 g angiocath

Stool for occult blood ☐

Medication Record

PRN

DiphenhydrAMINE 50 mg capsule i po q6h prn itching
Metoclopramide 10 mg IM po q6h prn N/V

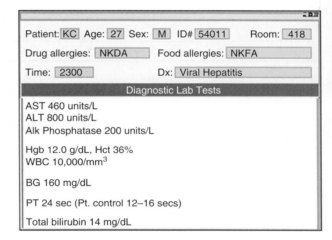

Patient: KC Age: 27 Sex: M ID# 54011 Room: 418
Drug allergies: NKDA Food allergies: NKFA
Time: 2300 Dx: Viral Hepatitis

Diagnostic Lab Tests

AST 460 units/L
ALT 800 units/L
Alk Phosphatase 200 units/L

Hgb 12.0 g/dL, Hct 36%
WBC 10,000/mm^3

BG 160 mg/dL

PT 24 sec (Pt. control 12–16 secs)

Total bilirubin 14 mg/dL

Collaborative Learning Activity: With a partner, **use the clinical situation and the electronic medical record** to:

1. Identify the pertinent patient information made known to you in the handoff *report*.	2. Identify the pertinent patient information made known to you from the *electronic medical record.*	3. Review the data in columns 1 and 2 and identify information that needs follow-up.

It is 2330. Prioritize your plan of care for the next hour:

Time	Plan of Care

The patient is diagnosed with hepatitis A and is tentatively scheduled for discharge in 2 days.

IP **1. Identify the discharge information that you would include in teaching the patient and his family how best to recover from hepatitis A.**

Diet:	Activity:
Fluids:	Skin care:
Nausea/vomiting:	Sexual concerns:
Preventing transmission:	Alcohol intake:
	Follow-up care:

Critical Reflection: To support patient-centered care and advocate teamwork and collaboration, write how you would discuss with the physician the IM order of metoclopramide:

_____

_____

_____

_____

3-12 PATIENT WITH PROSTATE CANCER AND MEDICATION ERROR

0700 Handoff Report:

> **S** Mr. T, 67 years old, has prostate cancer with metastasis to the bone. I have given him morphine IVP around the clock for pain, the last dose given at 0500. He is lethargic but responds when spoken to. He moans periodically and is mouth breathing so he needs frequent mouth care. His urine is amber. The 0600 vital signs are stable at T 99°F, P 76, R 18, BP 126/74. Intake is 100 mL, output is 150 mL. His wife spent the night in the room and is making arrangements for hospice care.

The following information is obtained from Mr. T's electronic medical record:

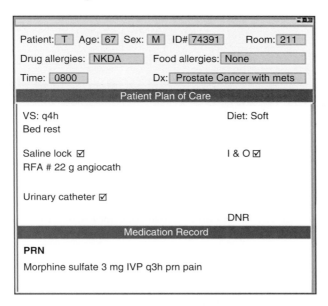

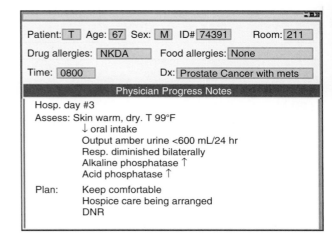

3 Critical Thinking Model Application

Collaborative Learning Activity: With a partner, **use the clinical situation and the electronic medical record** to:

1. Identify the pertinent patient information made known to you in the handoff *report*.	2. Identify the pertinent patient information made known to you from the *electronic medical record.*	3. Review the data in columns 1 and 2 and identify information that needs follow-up.

It is 0730. Prioritize your plan of care for the next hour:

Time	Plan of Care

1400 Mrs. T calls to inform you that Mr. T is in a lot of pain and she is very upset and tells you that the pain shots do not seem to be giving him any comfort. You call the physician and suggest an order for something stronger. The physician orders an additional 3 mg dose now to control the breakthrough pain. You administer hydromorphone 3 mg IVP at 1415. At 1430 Mrs. T calls you into the room and tells you that her husband is not breathing.

On assessment, you note that Mr. T has stopped breathing and there is no pulse.

1. Identify the nursing interventions that require immediate follow-up.	**2. Identify and discuss the ethical issue presented in this situation.**

Critical Reflection: To promote teamwork and collaboration, identify nursing interventions that would be beneficial for you and the family at this time:

_____

_____

_____

_____

_____

_____

_____

3-13 PATIENT WITH MASTECTOMY AND IV FLUID OVERLOAD

0700 Handoff Report:

 Mrs. S, 58 years old, is 1 day postop right radical mastectomy. Her dressing is clean and dry. She has a Hemovac that drained 50 mL. Her vital signs at 0600 are T 99.6°F, P 88, R 24, BP 150/90, pain level 3/10, pulse ox 95%. She is using the PCA and also has lactated Ringer's at 125 mL/hr. I started a new liter at 0600. Her right arm is elevated on a pillow; there is some swelling and she is complaining of some numbness.

The following information is obtained from Mrs. S's electronic medical record:

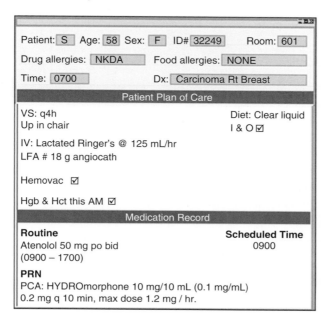

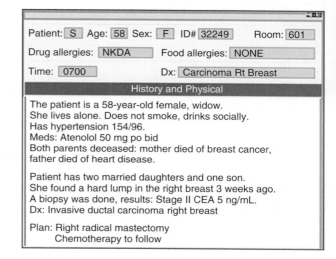

Collaborative Learning Activity: With a partner, **use the clinical situation and the electronic medical record** to:

1. Identify the pertinent patient information made known to you in the handoff *report*.	2. Identify the pertinent patient information made known to you from the *electronic medical record.*	3. Review the data in columns 1 and 2 and identify information that needs follow-up.

3 Critical Thinking Model Application

It is 0730. Prioritize your plan of care for the next hour:

Time	Plan of Care

0800: You assess the following on Mrs. S: Alert and oriented ×4. VS: T 99°F, P 94, R 28, BP 160/100. Lung sounds with crackles in the lower bases. Surgical dressing is clean and dry. Hemovac is compressed with 10 mL of reddish drainage. Right arm is elevated on a pillow. Fingers puffy, c/o a "numbness sensation." Stated on a 0 to 10 pain scale, the pain level is at 2. Abdominal sounds present ×4. Antiembolic hose on. Lactated Ringer's infusing, IV site without redness or swelling, 500 mL left.

1. Identify the nursing interventions that require immediate follow-up.	**2. Identify and discuss the postop educational needs of the patient.**

Critical Reflection: To provide patient-centered care, identify nursing interventions that would assist the patient in discussing the loss of her breast:

_____

_____

_____

_____

_____

_____

3-14 PATIENT WITH HF AND DIGOXIN TOXICITY

0700 Handoff Report:

 S Mr. S was admitted 2 days ago with heart failure. He had a restless night with some dyspnea and a dry nonproductive cough most of the night. Crackles are heard in both lungs. He has 3+ pitting edema in both legs and sacrum. His 0600 vital signs are T 97.6°F, P 110 and irregular, R 34, BP 150/100, pulse ox 94% with oxygen @ 3 L/min/NC. His IV site looks slightly puffy, but there is a good blood return. He denies pain but just started to complain of nausea. His serum K$^+$ this morning is 3.0 mEq. It might be low because he is retaining fluid. His physician always comes in early and the lab results are available.

The following information is obtained from Mr. S's electronic medical record:

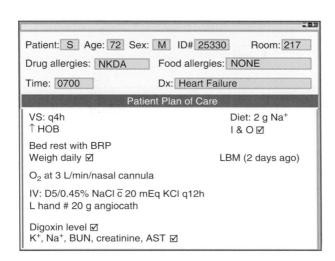

Patient: S   Age: 72   Sex: M   ID# 25330   Room: 217

Drug allergies: NKDA   Food allergies: NONE

Time: 0700   Dx: Heart Failure

Patient Plan of Care

VS: q4h   Diet: 2 g Na$^+$
↑ HOB   I & O ☑

Bed rest with BRP
Weigh daily ☑   LBM (2 days ago)

O$_2$ at 3 L/min/nasal cannula

IV: D5/0.45% NaCl c̄ 20 mEq KCl q12h
L hand # 20 g angiocath

Digoxin level ☑
K$^+$, Na$^+$, BUN, creatinine, AST ☑

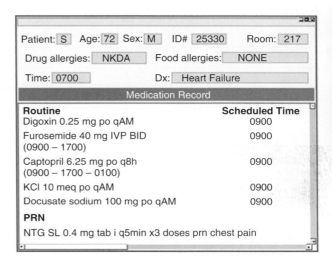

Patient: S   Age: 72 Sex: M   ID# 25330   Room: 217

Drug allergies: NKDA   Food allergies: NONE

Time: 0700   Dx: Heart Failure

Medication Record

Routine	Scheduled Time
Digoxin 0.25 mg po qAM	0900
Furosemide 40 mg IVP BID (0900 – 1700)	0900
Captopril 6.25 mg po q8h (0900 – 1700 – 0100)	0900
KCl 10 meq po qAM	0900
Docusate sodium 100 mg po qAM	0900
PRN	
NTG SL 0.4 mg tab i q5min x3 doses prn chest pain	

3 Critical Thinking Model Application

Collaborative Learning Activity: With a partner, **use the clinical situation and the electronic medical record** to:

1. Identify the pertinent patient information made known to you in the handoff *report*.	2. Identify the pertinent patient information made known to you from the *electronic medical record.*	3. Review the data in columns 1 and 2 and identify information that needs follow-up.

It is 0730. Prioritize your plan of care for the next hour:

Time	Plan of Care

0900: The physician has not come in to see Mr. S. Mr. S is alert but experiencing increasing shortness of breath, cough, and nausea and complaining of blurred vision. His pulse oximetry result is 88%. P 116 and irregular, R 34 and short and shallow, BP 152/100. Skin cool, color with slight cyanosis. Aside from the K⁺ of 3.0 mEq, Mr. S's Na⁺ is 135+ mEq, and his digoxin level is 2.4 ng/mL. You call the physician and learn that he is in surgery and will call you back within 30 minutes.

IP 1. Identify the nursing interventions that require immediate follow-up.	2. Write a nurse's note to describe the 0900 situation and the follow-up interventions.

Critical Reflection: To provide safe nursing care, identify how clinical reasoning was used to make a clinical decision.

_____

_____

_____

_____

_____

_____

_____

_____

3-15 PATIENT WITH HIP FRACTURE AND DVT

0700 Handoff Report:

 | Mrs. LV, 74 years old, is 4 days postop left hip fracture. She had a ConstaVac that was removed yesterday. Surgical dressing is clean and dry. Pedal pulse on the left foot is present and the circulation, movement, and sensation are within normal limits. Lung sounds with fine crackles at the lower bases in both lungs. You need to encourage her to deep breathe and use the incentive spirometer. Her 0600 vital signs are T 99.8°F, P 80, R 18, BP 130/82, pulse ox 96%. Pain level 7 at that time. She does not want to move, it seems like she is scared. I have given her acetaminophen two times during the night for leg pain, the last dose was at 0600. She is sleeping right now.

The following information is obtained from Mrs. LV's electronic medical record:

3 Critical Thinking Model Application

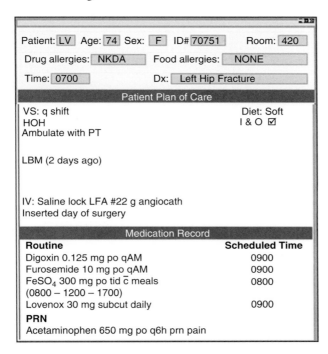

Patient: LV Age: 74 Sex: F ID# 70751 Room: 420
Drug allergies: NKDA Food allergies: NONE
Time: 0700 Dx: Left Hip Fracture

Patient Plan of Care

VS: q shift Diet: Soft
HOH I & O ☑
Ambulate with PT

LBM (2 days ago)

IV: Saline lock LFA #22 g angiocath
Inserted day of surgery

Medication Record

Routine	Scheduled Time
Digoxin 0.125 mg po qAM	0900
Furosemide 10 mg po qAM	0900
FeSO$_4$ 300 mg po tid c̄ meals (0800 – 1200 – 1700)	0800
Lovenox 30 mg subcut daily	0900
PRN	
Acetaminophen 650 mg po q6h prn pain	

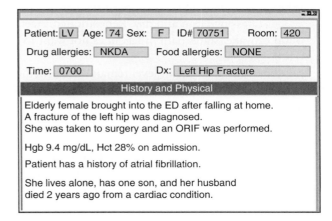

Patient: LV Age: 74 Sex: F ID# 70751 Room: 420
Drug allergies: NKDA Food allergies: NONE
Time: 0700 Dx: Left Hip Fracture

History and Physical

Elderly female brought into the ED after falling at home.
A fracture of the left hip was diagnosed.
She was taken to surgery and an ORIF was performed.

Hgb 9.4 mg/dL, Hct 28% on admission.

Patient has a history of atrial fibrillation.

She lives alone, has one son, and her husband
died 2 years ago from a cardiac condition.

Collaborative Learning Activity: With a partner, **use the clinical situation and the electronic medical record** to:

1. Identify the pertinent patient information made known to you in the handoff *report*.	2. Identify the pertinent patient information made known to you from the *electronic medical record.*	3. Review the data in columns 1 and 2 and identify information that needs follow-up.

It is 0730. Prioritize your plan of care for the next hour:

Time	Plan of Care

You review the nurse's notes from the night shift:

0000   Alert, moaning, states leg hurts, pain level 7. Circulation, movement, and sensation of left leg WNL. Dressing clean and dry. Repositioned. Acetaminophen given for pain.

0200   Awake, states pain in leg, does not want to be touched. Left pedal pulse palpable. Repositioned.

0400   Sleeping.

0600   C/o leg pain, pain level remains at 7. Medicated with acetaminophen.

You assess the following:

0730 Awake, alert, states "did not have a good night." Right leg pain level at 5. Left leg with pedal pulse, warm, cap. refill greater than 2 sec. Leg elevated on pillow. Dressing clean and dry. Right leg with weak pedal pulse, swelling and redness noted at calf and thigh. Tender to touch. Lung sounds with fine crackles, encouraged to take deep breaths. Bowel sounds present ×4, complaining of constipation.

IP	1. Identify the nursing interventions that require immediate follow-up.	2. Identify the instructions that you will give the nursing assistants at this time.

Critical Reflection: To promote safe nursing practice, the handoff report at 0700:

☐ communicated sufficient information to provide continuous care to the patient.

☐ lacked the following: _____

_____

3-16 PATIENT DIAGNOSED WITH PULMONARY EMBOLUS AND ON ANTICOAGULANT THERAPY

1500 Handoff Report:

S	Mrs. L was admitted with signs and symptoms of having developed a pulmonary embolus. She just had a baby 2 weeks ago. She has a heparin drip. The infusion pump is set at 20 mL/hr. You have 100 mL left. She slept well. Respirations are unlabored at 22. The right lower lung has diminished breath sounds. She will be started on Coumadin today. She is anxious to go home and be with her baby.

The following information is obtained from Mrs. L's electronic medical record:

Patient: L   Age: 32   Sex: F   ID# 06942   Room: 325

Drug allergies: NKDA   Food allergies: None

Time: 1500   Dx: Pulmonary Embolus

Patient Plan of Care

VS: q4h   Diet: Regular

Bed rest with BRP   I & O ☑

O_2 @ 3 L/min/NC prn SOB

IV: 500 mL D5W c̄ 20,000 units heparin
Infuse at 1000 units/hr
LFA #22 g angiocath

Daily PTT ☑   PT in AM ☐

Medication Record

Routine	Scheduled Time
Coumadin 2.5 mg po today at	1700
Coumadin 5 mg po at (0900)	0900

Coagulation Record

Date	PTT	Control	Heparin Dose
1st day	50 sec	25 sec	900 units/hr
2nd day	60 sec	25 sec	1000 units/hr
3rd day	90 sec	30 sec	1100 units/hr
Current	75 sec	30 sec	1000 units/hr

Collaborative Learning Activity: With a partner, **use the clinical situation and the electronic medical record** to:

1. Identify the pertinent patient information made known to you in the handoff *report*.	→	2. Identify the pertinent patient information made known to you from the *electronic medical record.*	→	3. Review the data in columns 1 and 2 and identify information that needs follow-up.

3 Critical Thinking Model Application

It is 1530. Prioritize your plan of care for the next hour:

Time	Plan of Care

1830 The nursing assistant informs you that the IV pump is beeping. You go in to assess the pump and you notice that the heparin bag is empty. You look at the infusion pump and it is set at 35 mL/hr instead of 25 mL/hr.

IP	1. Identify the nursing interventions that require immediate follow-up.	2. Document your findings as you would enter them in the electronic medical record.

Critical Reflection: To promote safe nursing practice, identify interventions that support the safe administration of heparin therapy and professional competency:

_____

_____

_____

_____

_____

3-17 PATIENT WITH SIGNS AND SYMPTOMS OF POSTOP COMPLICATIONS

1500 Handoff Report:

> **S** Ms. P, 23 years old, had an emergency appendectomy yesterday. She has Down syndrome. She has gotten up to the chair twice today. Surgical dressing is clean, dry, and intact. Bowel sounds are hypoactive. Her IV is infusing well; you have 200 mL left. Oral intake is 100 mL and output is 400 mL. I gave her morphine sulfate 8 mg IVP at noon for complaint of pain at a level of 8. Her noon vital signs are T 100°F, P 80, R 20, BP 110/78, pulse ox 98%.

The following information is obtained from Ms. P's electronic medical record:

Patient: P   Age: 23   Sex: F   ID# 58072   Room: 214

Drug allergies: NKDA   Food allergies: None

Time: 1500   Dx: Acute Appendicitis

Patient Plan of Care

VS: q4h   Diet: Clear liquid

Ambulate with assistance   I & O ☑

IV: 1 L D5/0.9% NaCl @ 125 mL/hr
LFA #22 g angiocath

Medication Record

Routine   **Scheduled Time**

Cefoxitin 1 g IVPB q8h   1800
(1000 – 1800 – 0200)

PRN

Morphine sulfate 8 mg IVP q4h prn pain
Metoclopramide 10 mg IVP q6h prn N/V

Intake and Output Record

7 – 3 shift:

Intake	Amt	Output	Time	Amt
Oral:	100	Void:	(0800)	50
			(0900)	50
			(1100)	75
			(1200)	50
			(1300)	75
			(1400)	100
IV:	900			
IVPB:	50	Emesis:	(1200)	100
Total:	1050			500

Collaborative Learning Activity: With a partner, **use the clinical situation and the electronic medical record** to:

1. Identify the pertinent patient information made known to you in the handoff *report*.	2. Identify the pertinent patient information made known to you from the *electronic medical record.*	3. Review the data in columns 1 and 2 and identify information that needs follow-up.

It is 1530. Prioritize your plan of care for the next hour:

Time	Plan of Care

2000 Ms. P's mother and family are at the bedside. They tell you that Ms. P is increasingly restless and is pulling at her surgical dressing. You note the following entries in the nursing notes:

Has voided a total of 100 mL since 1600. Emesis 100 mL greenish fluid at 1800, refused dinner. Morphine sulfate 8 mg and metoclopramide 10 mg given IVP at 1800.

IP	**1. Identify the nursing interventions that require immediate follow-up.**	**2. Identify a rationale for each nursing intervention that you plan to implement.**

Critical Reflection: To provide patient-centered care, identify nursing interventions that support the patient and family during this time:

_____

_____

_____

_____

3-18 PATIENT WITH CELLULITIS DEVELOPS ANGINA

0700 Handoff Report:

 S | Mr. O has cellulitis of the right leg. He is pretty much self-care and he says he is not used to being in bed so much. He stays in a chair most of the time with his leg elevated. His I & O is fine and his vital signs are stable at T 37°C, P 92, R 22, BP 164/94, pain level 0, pulse ox 98%. He has a dry dressing on the right leg and there is no drainage. His saline lock needs to be changed today and his fingerstick blood glucose was 110 this morning.

The following information is obtained from Mr. O's electronic medical record:

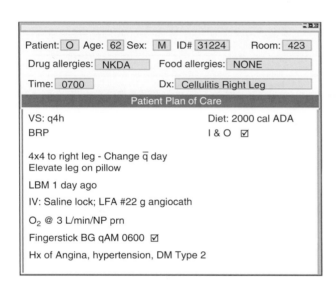

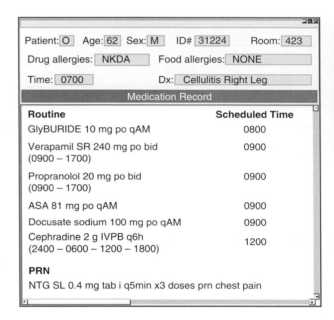

Collaborative Learning Activity: With a partner, **use the clinical situation and the electronic medical record** to:

1. Identify the pertinent patient information made known to you in the handoff *report*.	2. Identify the pertinent patient information made known to you from the *electronic medical record.*	3. Review the data in columns 1 and 2 and identify information that needs follow-up.

It is 0730. Prioritize your plan of care for the next hour:

Time	Plan of Care

1200: Mr. O returns to bed after having a BM. You note that he is short of breath and his skin is cool and clammy. You assess his vital signs, his radial pulse is 110 and irregular, respirations are 32, and his BP is 170/100. He tells you that he is feeling pressure on his chest. You assist him into bed and place him in high Fowler's position.

IP

1. Identify your follow-up nursing interventions.	2. Identify a rationale for each nursing intervention that you plan to implement.

Critical Reflection: To provide patient-centered care, identify nursing interventions that support the patient and family during this time:

_____

_____

_____

_____

3-19 PATIENT WITH TURP AND NS IRRIGATION

0700 Handoff Report:

> **S** "Mr. I, 70 years old, is 1 day postop TURP. He has a continuous 0.9% NaCl irrigation. I will hang up a new irrigation bag before I leave. He has had several clots during the shift. His vital signs are T 37.2°C, P 90, R 22, BP 160/93. He is alert and cheerful and told me that he leads a very active life. I gave him a suppository for c/o bladder spasms at 0500 this morning for a pain level of 7 out of 10. The IV was started at 0100 and it is behind since it slows down when the patient bends his arm."

The following information is obtained from Mr. I's electronic medical record:

Patient: I   Age: 70   Sex: M   ID# 02034   Room: 112

Drug allergies: NKDA   Food allergies: None

Time: 0700   Dx: BPH

Patient Plan of Care

VS q4h	Diet: Soft diet
Antiembolic hose on	LBM: On admission

IV: Lactated Ringer's at 75 mL/hr
#20 g angiocath RFA

3-way indwelling cath c̄ 30-mL balloon
0.9% NaCl cont irrigation - keep UA free of clots
Manual bladder irrigation with 0.9% NaCl prn

Medication Record

Routine   **Scheduled Time**
Docusate sodium 100 mg po daily   1000

PRN
Belladonna and opium supp. i q6h prn bladder
spasms

Intake and Output Record

11–7 shift:

	Intake	Output
Oral:	50	1300
	(NaCl irrigation	1000)
IV:	300	
Total:	350 mL	300 mL

---

3 Critical Thinking Model Application

 Collaborative Learning Activity: With a partner, **use the clinical situation and the electronic medical record** to:

1. Identify the pertinent patient information made known to you in the handoff *report.*	2. Identify the pertinent patient information made known to you from the *electronic medical record.*	3. Review the data in columns 1 and 2 and identify information that needs follow-up.

It is 0730. Prioritize your plan of care for the next hour:

Time	Plan of Care

0800: Mr. I is complaining of increased pain. He is grimacing, is diaphoretic, and tells you he has an urge to urinate. You note that the irrigation bag is empty and there are 50 mL of burgundy-colored urine in the urinary collection bag. There is urine leaking around the catheter.

1. Identify the nursing interventions that you would plan to implement immediately.	**2. Identify the follow-up nursing interventions for the rest of the shift.**

Critical Reflection: To promote safe nursing practice, the handoff report at 7:00 AM and the flowcharts:

☐ communicated sufficient information to provide continuous care to the patient.

☐ lacked the following: _____

_____

_____

_____

_____

_____

_____

3-20 PATIENT WITH TAH AND EPIDURAL CATHETER

0700 Handoff Report:

 "Mrs. HF, 46 years old, had a TAH-BSO yesterday. She had soft bowel sounds this morning. The abdominal dressing is clean and dry. Her peripheral IV is infusing well and she has an epidural infusion with fentanyl infusing through a pump. She has not had any breakthrough pain. The epidural dressing is intact and the catheter is fine. She has been mostly on bed rest, but she is to get up to a chair this morning. The 0600 vital signs are T 37.5°C, P 78, R 18, BP 130/80, pulse ox 98%. Her output was 500 mL."

The following information is obtained from Mrs. HF's electronic medical record:

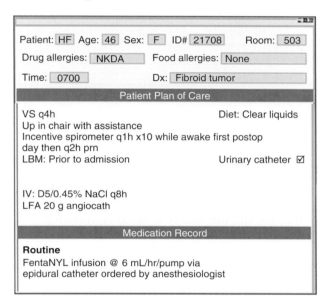

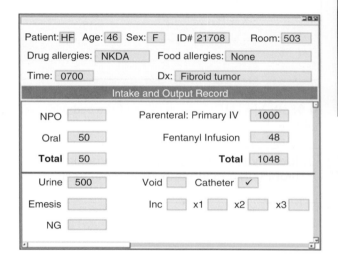

3 Critical Thinking Model Application

Collaborative Learning Activity: With a partner, **use the clinical situation and the electronic medical record** to:

1. Identify the pertinent patient information made known to you in the handoff *report*.	2. Identify the pertinent patient information made known to you from the *electronic medical record.*	3. Review the data in columns 1 and 2 and identify information that needs follow-up.

3 Critical Thinking Model Application

It is 0730. Prioritize your plan of care for the next hour:

Time	Plan of Care

At 0830: Mrs. HF sits at the side of the bed with assistance. Upon assessing the patient, you note that the tape holding the epidural line is no longer intact, the dressing is wet, and the epidural catheter is pulled out.

IP 1. Identify the nursing interventions that you would plan to implement immediately.	2. Document your findings as you would enter them in the electronic anecdotal nursing notes.

Critical Reflection: To provide patient-centered care, identify nursing interventions that support the patient during this time:

_____

_____

_____

_____

_____

_____

_____

3-21 CULTURALLY COMPETENT NURSING CARE

The nurse reviews the history and physical (H & P), the handoff report, and the day shift patient assessment.

Admitting Information: Mr. W, 72-year-old male of Chinese descent. Brought into the office by his son. The son provided most of the information because the patient speaks limited English. The patient lives in China but has been in the United States for 5 months visiting his son. He was planning to return home in a couple of weeks. Mr. W requests that the son be present and assist with questions during his physical examination.

Physical Examination:

Appearance: Small frame, thin man.

VS: T 101.8°F, P 92, R 28, BP 130/90, pulse oximetry 94%

Neuro: Alert, soft-spoken, smiles and answers questions appropriately via the son. PERRLA.

Resp: Crackles bilaterally. Productive cough with yellow-colored phlegm. Dyspnea. Indicates that "chest hurts all over."

CV: Pulse slightly irregular. Murmur—neg. Integ: Dry, decreased turgor.

GI: Abdomen soft, nontender. Son states his father is not eating very well. He misses the traditional cooking but does like some American soups. Denies constipation.

GU: No complaints. WNL.

Psychosocial: Quiet, widower.

Medications: Prescription medications—none. Has been using several herbal teas for "the cold in his chest."

Admitting Dx: Bilateral pneumonia

1500 Handoff Report: Mr. W has been in the hospital for 2 days. There is always someone in the room with the patient. His son spent the night with him. The patient is quiet and speaks limited English. He seems to respond better to male nurses. Lung sounds are still diminished in the lower bases. Has refused his bath for 2 days now. He has lost another pound since admission. His IV is infusing well at 125 mL/hr and Cefizox IVPB is ordered q12h.

Electronic entry by the day shift RN:

0800 Neuro: Awake, quiet, and cooperative. PERRLA.

Resp: Diminished in the lower bilateral bases. Productive cough with light yellowish sputum. Pulse ox 94%. O₂ at 2 L/min/NC. SOB noted on exertion.

CV/Skin: Warm, cap refill less than 3 sec. Turgor nonelastic.

GI: Active bowel sounds ×4 quadrants.

0900 GI: Ate 50% of breakfast. Family has brought in some food for the patient.

MS: Up to bathroom with assistance from the son. SOB noted on exertion. Son states that the father is upset because he believes his urine smells bad because of the IV medication.

1300 GI: Ate 10% of lunch. Drinking teas and soups brought from home.

1400: Systems unchanged.

3 Critical Thinking Model Application

Collaborative Learning Activity: With a partner, **use the clinical situation and the electronic medical record** to:

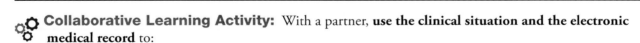

1. Identify the pertinent patient information made known to you from the H & P *report*.	2. Identify the pertinent patient information made known to you from the *handoff and assessments notes.*	3. Review the data in columns 1 and 2 and identify information that needs follow-up.

Use the **Cultural Considerations** listed in the left-hand side of the following box to develop **realistic nursing interventions** that demonstrate culturally sensitive care for Mr. W:

Cultural Considerations	Patient-centered Care
• Communication • Food preferences • View of health care practitioner role • Patient's role in the family • Patient's view of Western medicine with regard to current illness • Patient's view of what caused the illness • Patient's view of what would be beneficial for getting better	

On the third hospital day, Mr. W refuses the morning dose of Cefizox IVPB and refuses to let the nurse listen to his lungs. He tells the family that he is tired and wants to be left alone. His 0800 VS are T 99.9°F, P 96, R 26, BP 134/90, pulse oximetry 86%. Denies pain.

IP	1. Identify the nursing interventions that you would implement at this time.	2. Identify a rationale for each intervention that you plan to implement.

Critical Reflection: To provide patient-centered care, identify nursing interventions that support the patient and family during this time:

_____

_____

_____

_____

_____

_____

_____

3-22 PATIENT WITH ANTHRAX EXPOSURE

 S Mr. S, 46 years old, comes into the urgent care center with complaints of fatigue, muscle aches, a cough, and headache. Vital signs are T 99.8°F, P 90, R 28, BP 130/88. Pain level 0. Mr. S tells the nurse that he has had these symptoms for the last 48 hours and that he cannot afford to be ill. He says that he has a lot of work waiting for him at the office because there have been rumors regarding anthrax exposure of several people from one of the government buildings several blocks away.

The information obtained from Mr. S includes:

Examination	Familial History	Social History
Neuro: A & O c/o slight headache. Resp: Bilateral wheezing. Non-productive cough, SOB noted. C/o sore throat and chest area "a little sore." CV: Regular pulse, heart sounds WNL. GI: Anorexia. Abdomen soft, nontender. GU: WNL.	Married, 2 children, both healthy (1 male, 15 years; 1 female, 12 years). Wife works as a secretary part-time. Mother: Deceased; trauma from an auto accident. Father: DM type 2, hypertension. **Employment History:** Government employee for 15 years.	Alcohol: Drinks occasionally. Medications: Vitamins, echinacea tablets (heard it helped in decreasing the effects of a cold). Activities: Golfs twice a month, gym (weights and treadmill). Describes himself as a "generally healthy person."

3 Critical Thinking Model Application

Collaborative Learning Activity: With a partner, **use the clinical situation and the information obtained** to:

1. Identify the pertinent patient information made known to you in the *report*.	2. Identify the pertinent patient information made known to you from the *information provided*.	3. Review the data in columns 1 and 2 and identify information that needs follow-up.

The patient is diagnosed and admitted to the acute care setting with signs and symptoms of inhalation anthrax. Read the following **physician orders** and **write a rationale** for each order:

Physician Orders	
1. Standard precautions 2. Chest x-ray stat 3. VS q4h with neuro checks 4. CBC, 12-chem panel, UA 5. Ciprofloxacin 400 mg IVPB now	1. Standard precautions: _____ _____ _____ _____ _____ _____ 2. Chest x-ray stat: _____ _____ _____ _____ 3. VS q4h with neuro checks: _____ _____ _____ 4. CBC, 12-chem panel, UA: _____ _____ 5. Ciprofloxacin 400 mg IVPB now: _____ _____ _____

At 1600 the nursing assistant reports the following: T 99°F, P 120, R 30, BP 118/80, pulse oximetry 92%. The patient was difficult to arouse.

1. Identify the nursing interventions that you would plan to implement immediately.	2. Identify a rationale for each nursing intervention that you plan to implement.

Critical Reflection: To provide patient-centered care, identify nursing interventions that support the patient and family during this time:

_____
_____
_____
_____
_____
_____

SECTION 4

Management and Leadership

4-1 MENTORING AND NURSING MANAGEMENT

The supervisor of a medical unit has recently hired several new RNs just out of nursing school. Two of the new RNs have started on the day shift. As an RN with 7 years of experience, you have been assigned to orient and precept one of the new RNs. The new RN will work with you for 3 months.

Information about the experienced RN: You have worked mainly on the medical unit and are considered an expert. You are always on time. You are organized and can be counted on "to get the job done." You are frequently given all the new employees to orient. You have never complained and you like working with nurses, but you are getting pretty tired of having to be the one that is assigned to orient the new employees all the time.

Information about the new RN: He is in his twenties, quiet but friendly. He works steadily, has a good knowledge base, but has difficulty asking questions. He has managed the care of three patients in school. He was late the first day on the unit and tells the nurse that he "is more of a night person."

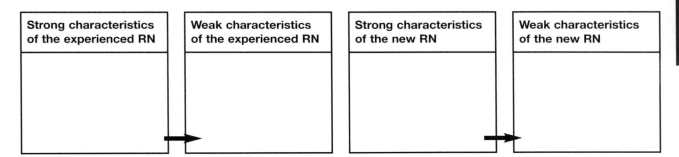

1. Identify the strong and weak characteristics demonstrated in the RNs.

Strong characteristics of the experienced RN	Weak characteristics of the experienced RN	Strong characteristics of the new RN	Weak characteristics of the new RN

2. Prioritize the one major issue that may cause conflict initially.

1. _____
   _____
   _____

As the experienced RN, how would you handle this major issue?
_____
_____

Before implementing the plan, what other issues should be considered?
_____
_____

4 Management and Leadership

As the experienced nurse, you develop the following goals to help guide the progress of the new RN. You discuss these goals with the new RN.

Goals for the First Week	Goals for the Second Week

At the end of the 2 weeks, the new RN has not been able to achieve the set goals. The experienced RN sets up a time to meet with the new RN. During the meeting, the new RN is visibly upset.

> **1. Identify the issues that may be affecting the new RN.**

Issues:
_____
_____
_____
_____
_____
_____

With a partner, role-play the part of the experienced nurse and the new RN.

As the experienced RN, how would you handle this situation?	As the new RN, how would you like this situation handled?

4-2 WORKING THROUGH THE CHANGE PROCESS

The hospital administration has agreed to replace all white board patient communication boards with the first electronic patient communication board. The new boards will initially be installed in every patient room of the medical-surgical units. For the last 3 months the staff has been required to attend computer training classes to learn how to input and update data from the main computer onto the electronic patient communication board. The information on the electronic patient communication board needs to be verified every shift and updated as new orders are received. Training manuals and informational flyers have been developed.

Information about administration's decision: The electronic patient communication board offers more flexibility to immediately update information from the main computer onto the electronic patient communication board. The electronic patient communication board has the upgraded feature of automatically translating selected information into six different languages with just one click. Charge nurses and staff nurses from all shifts have been involved in evaluating and giving feedback. Administration has invested time and money into this new electronic patient communication board, is excited about the other patient-centered features that can be developed, and is committed to installing this throughout the hospital. The staff will have the opportunity to provide feedback after 3 months of use.

Information about the nursing staff: The implementation of the new electronic patient communication board has brought about mixed feelings among the nursing staff.

Comments from the nurses range from "The white board is so much easier to keep up," "Some patients, such as the elderly, cannot even read the information on the board," "It is a useless piece of technology and is one more required task for us to do," to "I am excited to see how patients react when they are able to see us update the information in their language." The managers, supervisors, and charge nurses are asked to support this change and to ensure that all nursing staff follow through every shift.

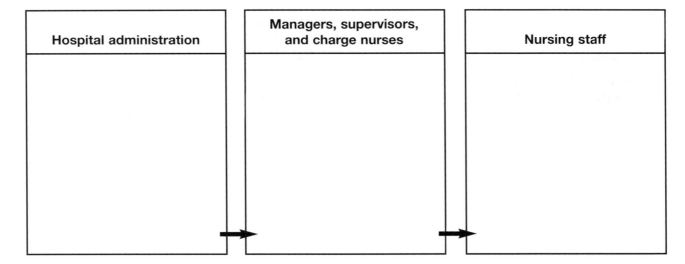

1. **Identify the issues/reactions from the different levels.**

Hospital administration	Managers, supervisors, and charge nurses	Nursing staff

How does the implementation of the electronic patient communication board and the nursing staff's comments and feelings correlate with the change process?

_____

_____

_____

You are the charge nurse of the unit that has been selected to be the first one to use the new patient communication board. Some nurses are very excited to be the first ones to use the program and other nurses are requesting to transfer to another unit. Administration has asked you to ensure that all nursing staff use the patient communication board and to identify how the administrative staff can help you facilitate the implementation of this electronic communication board on your unit.

1. Identify helpful strategies that support the implementation and help your staff cope with the change.	2. Identify specific requests that can guide administration in helping you and your staff implement this change.

How does the development of **helpful strategies,** both for the nursing staff and for administration, help with the process of change?

_____

_____

_____

After 2 weeks of using the program, your most experienced nurse complains about the additional work and how the patients are not even interested in the electronic communication board, She says that she does not see any benefit in this change. You, as the charge nurse, know that all the units will be using the electronic communication board within the next 6 months. The nurse is very good and you want to support her.

As the charge nurse, how would you handle this situation?	As the nurse, how would you like this situation handled?

4-3 TEAMWORK AND DELEGATION

An RN is transferred to the medical unit after working 5 years in the intensive care unit. It has taken some time—3 months to be exact—to organize and manage the care of 4 to 5 patients assigned to her on the day shift. The patients on the medical unit are high acuity and have multiple problems. Most of the staff has been very supportive, always checking to see whether they can help. However, the RN has observed one nursing assistant who rarely helps out the other staff members. The RN also believes that some interventions that the nursing assistant has done have been performed incorrectly.

Information about the RN: The RN is used to working independently. She would rather do the procedure or provide the care herself to ensure that it is done correctly. This has been a difficult transition for her because she has to rely on ancillary help to complete her work. Although the RN can delegate many tasks, she finds herself avoiding this nursing assistant and mostly doing the tasks herself. She stays late every day to complete the documentation on the patients.

Information about the nursing assistant: The nursing assistant has been on this unit for 1 year. She feels pretty comfortable with her skills and has even shown other nursing assistants how to take short cuts. She enjoys working by herself and takes pride in not asking anyone for help. She does not like being told how to do something that she already knows how to do. She is frustrated with the RN because the RN seems to be running around in circles. As far as she is concerned, she will do her job, and, unless asked, she will not do anything extra.

> 1. **Identify the characteristics demonstrated in the RN that interfere with effective delegation.**
>
> _____
> _____
> _____
> _____
> _____
> _____
> _____
> _____
> _____
> _____

In managing this situation, what can the RN do to create a more conducive working environment with the nursing assistant?

_____

_____

_____

The following day the nursing assistant is assigned to work with the RN. There are numerous tasks that need to be done for the patients. The nurse has the following tasks that need to be done for the assigned patients: vital signs, three bed baths, assessments, saline lock flushes, emptying urinary collection bags on two patients, emptying a J-P device, sterile dressing change, passing narcotic medications, monitoring IV fluids, NG tube bolus feeding, oral suctioning, deep suctioning, pulse oximetry, and starting oxygen per nasal cannula.

1. List the tasks that need to be performed by the RN.	2. List the tasks that may be delegated to the nursing assistant.

List the criteria that should be considered before delegating a task to another person.

_____

_____

_____

After the RN has taken her own noon vital signs, the nursing assistant approaches her and asks her why she did not let her take the noon vitals on the patients.

With a partner, role-play the part of the RN and the nursing assistant.

As the RN, how would you problem-solve this situation?	As the nursing assistant, what would you like to come out of this situation?

4-4 PRACTICE AND ETHICAL ISSUE

Two RNs have worked the day shift together on the oncology unit for several years. Both are expert nurses and through the years they have become close personal friends. RN Nurse A has accepted the position of charge nurse of the oncology unit, and RN Nurse B continues as a staff nurse. For the last 6 months, the charge nurse has been concerned about numerous discrepancies in the narcotic count. Lately, an increasing number of patients have been complaining that they are not obtaining pain relief after being medicated. After a careful investigation by the administrative staff, it was noted that all the narcotic count discrepancies occurred on the day shift. RN Nurse A, the charge nurse, is the only person informed of the current findings. A follow-up investigation will be conducted.

Information about RN Nurse A: The RN is married and has two children. She is frequently involved with the school activities of the children. She loves the staff and enjoys her work but is still learning the duties of a manager. She has a difficult time supervising and evaluating staff and seems to avoid handling any conflict situations. She has noticed that RN Nurse B has been irritable but has assumed that her recent marital separation is contributing to her behavior. After assessing the behavior of RN Nurse B, she is wondering whether her friend may be involved with the narcotic discrepancies.

Information about RN Nurse B: The RN has two children in school and has recently separated from her husband. She has been unable to be active in her children's school activities because of the added demands brought on by the separation. She has been suffering from migraine headaches but cannot afford to miss any work because the couple had just purchased a new home before the separation. She has asked RN Nurse A to assign her to extra shifts or overtime whenever possible.

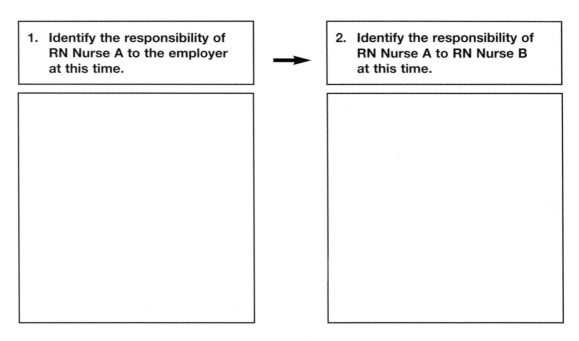

1. Identify the responsibility of RN Nurse A to the employer at this time.

2. Identify the responsibility of RN Nurse A to RN Nurse B at this time.

RN Nurse A feels that she is not being honest with the staff by not sharing the administrative decision to conduct a preliminary investigation. Identify issues that should be considered in this situation.

_____

_____

_____

For 3 weeks the narcotic count has been correct. Today, RN Nurse B is assigned to a terminally ill patient. She is preparing to administer pain medication to a patient and takes a syringe labeled morphine sulfate 10 mg from the narcotic drawer. She administers the medication IV to the patient. Thirty minutes later the patient is moaning with pain, and the family is very upset seeing him in such pain. The physician is called, and an order for a stat dose of morphine sulfate 5 mg IV is given. RN Nurse A administers the drug to the patient because RN Nurse B is at lunch. The patient is calm for the next 2 hours. RN Nurse A informs RN Nurse B about the additional dose of pain medication given to the patient. At the end of the shift, there is a discrepancy with the morphine sulfate and the narcotic count.

1. Identify the responsibility of RN Nurse A to the employer at this time.	2. Identify the responsibility of RN Nurse A to RN Nurse B at this time.

The next day, RN Nurse B is again preparing to administer morphine sulfate 10 mg IV push to the patient. RN Nurse B emptied the contents of the morphine sulfate into another syringe and put this syringe in her pocket. She then filled the current syringe with saline solution and took this syringe into the room and gave the saline solution to the patient.

RN Nurse A noticed that RN Nurse B had a syringe with liquid in her pocket as she was going home. RN Nurse A confronts RN Nurse B. RN Nurse B tells her friend that it is saline solution, but she refuses to discard it or to give it to RN Nurse A. With a partner, role-play the part of RN Nurse A and RN Nurse B.

As RN Nurse A, identify the outcome of RN Nurse B's action.	Identify the professional responsibility of RN Nurse A.

As RN Nurse B, what would you like to come out of this situation?

4-5 TEAMWORK AND COLLABORATION

The RN works on an endocrine unit in a hospital that uses a team approach to deliver patient care. The team consists of an RN, an LVN, and two nursing assistants. The RN is responsible for the supervision and the delegation of care. A new, highly recommended LVN has recently been hired to work on the unit. During the first week of orientation, the supervising RN noticed that the LVN was friendly but did not check the insulin dosages with anyone before giving the insulin injections to the patients. The RN told the LVN to have all insulin dosages double-checked before giving. The LVN told one of the nursing assistants that the RN did not trust her. Later, the RN again saw the LVN giving an insulin injection to another patient without checking the insulin dose. The RN questioned the LVN, and the LVN responded that she forgot because she never had to have her work checked in her previous job and she would remember to double-check the dose next time.

Information about the RN: The RN has been working on the endocrine unit for 2 years. She is very conscientious, and, because she has diabetes mellitus, she takes a special interest in working with patients who have diabetes. She works closely with her staff and has not had any serious staff problems. She can tell that the LVN has a lot of experience and feels a little intimidated by her at times. The RN has little patience for what she considers "unsafe practice" behaviors.

Information about the LVN: The LVN has been a nurse for 15 years and is recognized for providing good patient care. She has worked in several hospitals. In her last job, she worked in a skilled nursing facility where she had increased responsibility. She decided to return to the acute care setting because it offered better financial benefits. She feels that she has a lot of experience and is more familiar with some clinical situations than the newly graduated RNs. She can tell that the staff RN is recently out of school.

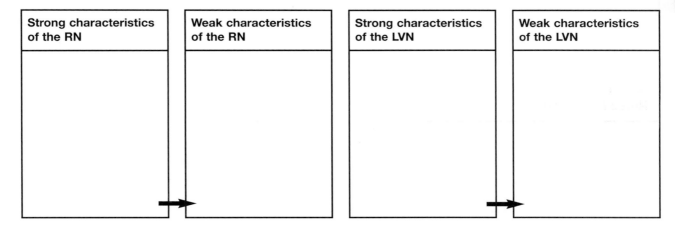

1. Identify the strong and weak characteristics demonstrated in each nurse.

Strong characteristics of the RN	Weak characteristics of the RN	Strong characteristics of the LVN	Weak characteristics of the LVN

IP 2. Prioritize the major issue that needs to be addressed at this time.

1. _____
   _____
   _____

As the RN, how would you handle this situation?

_____
_____
_____
_____

For the next 2 weeks, the RN noticed that the LVN had been double-checking the insulin dosages. Today, the unit is very busy and one patient in particular is very upset and requested to speak with the RN. The patient complained of several things but was especially upset because he was going to receive the wrong dose of insulin this morning. The patient explained that he asked the LVN how much insulin she was giving him and that she said 10 units of NPH. The patient insisted that he normally was given 12 units of NPH every morning. The LVN checked and the patient was correct.

The RN discussed the patient's comments with the LVN. The LVN agreed with the patient's comments, telling the RN that because the 10 units of NPH was less than the ordered dose, it was easily corrected. The RN decided to set up a meeting with the LVN to discuss the incident further and to present the following anecdotal note:

12/31 0900 Patient X complained that the LVN was going to administer 10 units of NPH insulin to him this morning instead of the ordered NPH 12 units. The LVN rechecked the ordered amount and proceeded to administer the correct dose to the patient.

I have told the LVN to double-check all insulin dosages before administering the injection to the patients. The LVN does not realize the seriousness of this behavior.

Discuss, evaluate, and rewrite the anecdotal note.

Anecdotal notes should contain:

The RN meets with the LVN.

With a partner, role-play the part of the RN and the LVN.

As the RN, how would you handle this situation?	**Identify key points to keep in mind when conducting an evaluation meeting with an employee.**
_____	
_____	_____
_____	_____
_____	_____
_____	_____
_____	_____
_____	_____
_____	_____
_____	_____

4-6 ADVOCATING CULTURAL COMPETENCY AND SENSITIVITY

The medical unit staff of an acute care hospital includes several RNs who have worked on this unit for more than 10 years. In addition to caring for high-acuity patients, the nurses on the medical unit have also seen a change in the cultural makeup of the staff. The hospital has recently hired six new RNs from various ethnic backgrounds: two Middle Eastern nurses, one Chinese nurse, one Korean nurse, one Hispanic nurse, and one male nurse from Nigeria. All the nurses were trained outside the United States and were successful in passing the NCLEX-RN examination. Although all the nurses have taken additional classes and training, this is their first full-time job in the acute care setting.

After going through the regular hospital orientation, the nurses are assigned to work on the day and evening shifts. After 2 months, three of the female nurses are having great difficulty working on the medical unit. Several of the regular RNs are complaining that the new nurses are not as competent and that they do not know how to relate with the staff and with the patients. Several staff members have asked to be transferred to another unit.

The unit manager solicited input from the new RNs and the regular staff and was told the following:

Comments made from the new RNs:
- Do not feel they are viewed as competent RNs.
- Staff members are impatient with them and take over tasks instead of letting them learn the tasks.
- Unlicensed personnel do not come to them with patient problems.
- General comments are made that make them feel incompetent.
- Have even been told to "speak English" several times.
- Their names have been changed to names that the staff can easily pronounce.
- There are a couple of RNs and staff members who are sympathetic and helpful.

Comments made from the regular RNs and staff:
- Handoff reports are difficult to understand.
- Interactions with patients are minimal and not personal.
- They require a lot of guidance and leave many tasks for the other shifts.
- New RNs are afraid to approach physicians or to call physicians for orders.

1. List the primary issues as viewed by the new RNs.

2. List the primary issues as viewed by the regular RNs and staff.

Analyze the issues presented and list the management and cultural issues that need to be addressed.

Management-Related Issues/Needs	Culturally Related Issues/Needs

List management strategies that should be considered to address the issues presented:

_____

_____

_____

_____

_____

_____

_____

In the clinical setting, it is important to become aware of cultural communication (tone of voice, use of words, gestures, touch, nonverbal communication) with staff and peers.

With a partner, identify cultural beliefs and values seen among peers and staff in the clinical setting. Discuss clinical examples and the implications related to health care delivery.

Possible cultural beliefs and values:

4-7 RECOGNIZING AND DEALING WITH INCIVILITY

The registry RN routinely accepts nursing assignments in a well-known medical center. She enjoys working on the surgical units but usually turns down assignments if asked to work in the endocrine unit. It is rumored that the endocrine unit is the least desired unit to work on. Not only are the patients highly acute but the staff lacks the spirit of teamwork and collaboration. Administration has noticed that the endocrine unit has the highest staff turnover of any unit in the hospital.

Today, the registry RN accepted to work on the surgical unit but upon arriving to the medical center, she is asked to work on the endocrine unit since they are very short of staff. She agrees since she has already reported to work.

Information about the shift experience: At the end of the shift the registry RN is very upset and discusses her experience with the unit supervisor. She relates the following:

"Upon arrival to the unit, I am assigned to 4 highly acute patients (2 unstable diabetic patients, 1 patient with acute pancreatitis, and one patient with a heparin infusion for a DVT).

The registry RN shared the following concerns:
- She discussed her assignment with the charge nurse shortly after reviewing her assignment because of the numerous medications that needed to be administered to each of the patients. The charge nurse informed her that the other nurses had been assigned the patients they had the previous day and they all had 4 and some even 5 patients. She was told that she was an experienced RN and that she should be able to handle the patients.

- She asked for help and one RN told her that she had her own assignment and not to ask her for help. She overheard this same RN tell the charge nurse how registry nurses are slow and incompetent.

- One of her patients began to show signs of hypoglycemia and she asked a staff RN to help her obtain a fingerstick blood glucose. The RN rolled her eyes and reluctantly did the fingerstick blood glucose. After giving her the glucose results, the staff RN said she was late for her lunch and left.

1. Identify behaviors experienced by the registry nurse that demonstrate incivility and increase the risk of patient safety.

_____
_____
_____
_____
_____
_____

4 Management and Leadership

The registry RN indicated that she will refuse any future assignments to the endocrine unit and wants to file a complaint. The supervisor advises that the first step of discussing her concerns is now taking place and that a formal written complaint is not necessary. She assures the registry nurse that she will speak to the charge nurse on the endocrine unit and that she will make sure that the registry nurse is not assigned to the endocrine unit in the future.

2. Evaluate the unit supervisor's response and the suggested follow up with the unit charge nurse.	3. List organizational strategies that create awareness of incivility and zero tolerance for these types of behavior.
 • _____ • _____ • _____ • _____ • _____ • _____ • _____	 • _____ • _____ • _____ • _____ • _____ • _____ • _____

Access the American Nurses Association Position Statement: Incivility, Bullying, and Workplace Violence, July 22, 2015 (http://www.nursingworld.org).

List behaviors and actions that <u>promote incivility</u> in the workplace:

• _____

• _____

• _____

• _____

• _____

⚠ With a partner use the American Nurses Association Position Statement: Incivility, Bullying, and Workplace Violence or other resources to identify how best to prepare and prevent incivility in the workplace and **create a culture of respect and safety.**

Create a culture of respect and safety:
_____ _____ _____ _____ _____ _____ _____

SECTION 5

NCLEX Examination Preparation

5-1 NCLEX EXAMINATION PREPARATION #1

INSTRUCTIONS: Circle the best answer(s) for each test question. Write your rationale for selecting the answer. To enhance your learning and test-taking skills, discuss your answer and rationale with a partner. The answer and the rationale can be found on the back of this page.

1. The nurse is demonstrating how to minimize occlusion of a feeding tube when administering medications. Which nursing intervention is most important to include in the demonstration?
   a. Withdraw any residual, give the medication, and flush with 30 mL of water.
   b. Flush the tube with 30 mL of water before and after giving the medication.
   c. Use 30 mL of lukewarm water to flush the tube after giving the medication.
   d. Inject 15 mL of air before and after giving the medication.

   Rationale: _____
   _____
   _____
   _____
   _____

2. The nurse is assigned to a patient admitted today with the diagnosis of paralytic ileus. In caring for the patient, the nurse expects to find the following on the patient (Select all that apply.):
   a. Hypotension
   b. Abdominal distention
   c. Clear liquid diet
   d. Decreased or absent bowel sounds
   e. Passing small amounts of tarry stool

   Rationale: _____
   _____
   _____
   _____
   _____

3. The client is receiving total parenteral nutrition through a single-lumen central catheter by infusion pump. Vancomycin 0.5 g in 100 mL 0.9% Sodium Chloride is ordered daily IVPB. To safely administer this IVPB, the nurse plans to
   a. administer the IVPB through a Y-port tubing above the infusion pump.
   b. stop the total parenteral nutrition infusion for 30 minutes to infuse the IVPB.
   c. start a peripheral line for the IVPB.
   d. use a mini-drip tubing for the IVPB.

   Rationale: _____
   _____
   _____
   _____
   _____

ANSWER KEY FOR NCLEX EXAMINATION PREPARATION #1

HELPFUL HINTS: Read all test questions carefully. Identify key words in the question that will guide you in answering the question. In these test questions the **key words** to consider are **"most important"** and **"safely."** Consider carefully all options in the "Select all that apply" questions. Compare your rationale with the one in the test question.

1. The nurse is demonstrating how to minimize occlusion of a feeding tube when administering medications. Which nursing intervention is most important to include in the demonstration?
   a. Withdraw any residual, give the medication, and flush with 30 mL of water.
   b. Flush the tube with 30 mL of water before and after giving the medication.
   c. Use 30 mL of lukewarm water to flush the tube after giving the medication.
   d. Inject 15 mL of air before and after giving the medication.

   Rationale: The answer is (b). It is important to check the patency of the feeding tube before the administration of medications. Flushing the feeding tube after medication administration helps to clear the feeding tube. Options (a), (c), and (d) do not present the proper technique for administering medications through a feeding tube.

2. The nurse is assigned to a patient admitted today with the diagnosis of paralytic ileus. In caring for the patient, the nurse expects to find the following on the patient (Select all that apply.):
   a. Hypotension
   b. Abdominal distention
   c. Clear liquid diet
   d. Decreased or absent bowel sounds
   e. Passing small amounts of tarry stool

   Rationale: The answers are (b) and (d). Option (b), distention, occurs as intestinal contents accumulate in the intestine and are not pushed forward down the intestine. Option (d) is correct because peristalsis is decreased or absent as the obstruction progresses. Option (a), hypotension, is not an expected finding. Option (c), a clear liquid diet, is usually ordered when the bowel sounds begin to return after the paralytic ileus. Option (e), passing tarry stools, is not common in the patient experiencing a paralytic ileus.

3. The client is receiving total parenteral nutrition through a single-lumen central catheter by infusion pump. Vancomycin 0.5 g in 100 mL 0.9% Sodium Chloride is ordered daily IVPB. To safely administer this IVPB, the nurse plans to
   a. administer the IVPB through a Y-port tubing above the infusion pump.
   b. stop the total parenteral nutrition infusion for 30 minutes to infuse the IVPB.
   c. start a peripheral line for the IVPB.
   d. use a mini-drip tubing for the IVPB.

   Rationale: The answer is (c). The IVPB should be administered via a separate IV line. Option (a) does not safely administer the IVPB because the total parenteral nutrition is continuously being infused. Option (b) indicates stopping the total parenteral nutrition, which may initiate a hypoglycemic reaction. Option (d) can be used but does not identify where the IVPB will be administered.

5-2 NCLEX EXAMINATION PREPARATION #2

INSTRUCTIONS: Circle the one best answer for each test question. Write your rationale for selecting the answer. To enhance your learning and test-taking skills, discuss your answer and rationale with a partner. The answer and the rationale can be found on the back of this page.

1. The nurse learns in report that the serum potassium level of a client is 5.5 mEq/L this morning. The client's physician is in surgery, so a message is left at the physician's office. The client is on the following medications at 0800: famotidine 20 mg po and spironolactone 50 mg po. Which action by the nurse is most appropriate?
   a. Hold the morning dose of famotidine until the physician returns the call.
   b. Hold the morning dose of spironolactone until the physician returns the call.
   c. Hold all the morning medications until the physician returns the call.
   d. Give all the morning medications as ordered.

   Rationale: _____
   _____
   _____
   _____
   _____

2. The nurse is caring for a client with diabetes mellitus type 2. The following medications are listed on the client's medication record: metformin 0.5 g po bid and repaglinide 1 mg po 30 minutes a.c. meals. The morning blood glucose fingerstick is 98 mg/dL. Which action by the nurse is most appropriate?
   a. Hold the morning po medications.
   b. Give the metformin but hold the repaglinide.
   c. Give the repaglinide but hold the metformin.
   d. Give the po medications as ordered.

   Rationale: _____
   _____
   _____
   _____
   _____

3. The client with end-stage renal disease is scheduled for hemodialysis in 2 hours. He has an (L) AV fistula and needs assistance with feeding. In delegating the care of the client to the certified nursing assistant, which nursing order is of priority?
   a. Feed the client first.
   b. Give all morning care before the dialysis.
   c. Take the blood pressure in the right arm.
   d. Gently feel for the thrill on the left arm.

   Rationale: _____
   _____
   _____
   _____
   _____

5 NCLEX Examination Preparation

ANSWER KEY FOR NCLEX EXAMINATION PREPARATION #2

HELPFUL HINTS: Read all test questions carefully. Identify key words in the question that will guide you in answering the question. In these test questions the **key words** to consider are **"most appropriate"** and **"priority."** Compare your rationale with the one in the test question.

1. The nurse learns in report that the serum potassium level of a client is 5.5 mEq/L this morning. The client's physician is in surgery, so a message is left at the physician's office. The client is on the following medications at 0800: famotidine 20 mg po and spironolactone 50 mg po. Which action by the nurse is most appropriate?
   a. Hold the morning dose of famotidine until the physician returns the call.
   b. Hold the morning dose of spironolactone until the physician returns the call.
   c. Hold all the morning medications until the physician returns the call.
   d. Give all the morning medications as ordered.

   Rationale: The answer is (b). Spironolactone is a potassium-sparing diuretic. Because the morning serum K+ level is high, the drug should be held until further orders are obtained from the physician. Option (a) does not affect the potassium level. Options (c) and (d) do not correlate the effects of the specific drugs to the electrolyte value.

2. The nurse is caring for a client with diabetes mellitus type 2. The following medications are listed on the client's medication record: metformin 0.5 g po bid and repaglinide 1 mg po 30 minutes a.c. meals. The morning blood glucose fingerstick is 98 mg/dL. Which action by the nurse is most appropriate?
   a. Hold the morning po medications.
   b. Give the metformin but hold the repaglinide.
   c. Give the repaglinide but hold the metformin.
   d. Give the po medications as ordered.

   Rationale: The answer is (d). The morning fingerstick result is within normal limits. Drug therapy should continue as ordered to maintain the blood glucose within normal limits. Options (a), (b), and (c) would not help the client remain in glycemic control.

3. The client with end-stage renal disease is scheduled for hemodialysis in 2 hours. He has an (L) AV fistula and needs assistance with feeding. In delegating the care of the client to the certified nursing assistant, which nursing order is of priority?
   a. Feed the client first.
   b. Give all morning care before the dialysis.
   c. Take the blood pressure in the right arm.
   d. Gently feel for the thrill on the left arm.

   Rationale: The answer is (c). The AV fistula is the vascular access for the hemodialysis. Care must be taken not to occlude or cause trauma to the site. Options (a) and (b) are important but not the priority nursing order. Option (d) is part of the assessment process that is the responsibility of the professional nurse and should not be delegated.

5-3 NCLEX EXAMINATION PREPARATION #3

INSTRUCTIONS: Circle the one best answer for each test question. Write your rationale for selecting the answer. To enhance your learning and test-taking skills, discuss your answer and rationale with a partner. The answer and the rationale can be found on the back of this page.

1. At 1000 the nurse realizes that clonidine 0.1 mg po was administered to the wrong client at 0900. Which nursing action is of priority?
   a. Fill out an incident report.
   b. Notify the physician.
   c. Take the client's blood pressure.
   d. Take the vital signs of the client at noon.

   Rationale: _____
   _____
   _____
   _____
   _____

2. A beta-blocking agent is added to the pharmacologic therapy of a client with heart failure. An expected therapeutic effect is:
   a. a decrease in complaints of fatigue.
   b. a decrease in the heart rate.
   c. an increase in blood pressure.
   d. an increase in diuresis.

   Rationale: _____
   _____
   _____
   _____
   _____

3. The client is taking hydrochlorothiazide 25 mg po daily and is started on the ACE inhibitor lisinopril 10 mg po daily. Which nursing intervention indicates the most appropriate follow-through action?
   a. Monitor the client's output.
   b. Assess the client for impaired skin integrity.
   c. Assess the client's cardiac rhythm.
   d. Monitor the client's blood pressure.

   Rationale: _____
   _____
   _____
   _____
   _____

5 NCLEX Examination Preparation

ANSWER KEY FOR NCLEX EXAMINATION PREPARATION #3

HELPFUL HINTS: Read all test questions carefully. Identify key words in the question that will guide you in answering the question. In these test questions the **key words** to consider are **"priority,"** **"expected therapeutic effect,"** and **"most appropriate."** Compare your rationale with the one in the test question.

1. At 1000 the nurse realizes that clonidine 0.1 mg po was administered to the wrong client at 0900. Which nursing action is of priority?
   a. Fill out an incident report.
   b. Notify the physician.
   (c.) Take the client's blood pressure.
   d. Take the vital signs of the client at noon.

   Rationale: The answer is (c). Clonidine is an alpha-adrenergic agonist and blocking agent. After oral administration, clonidine begins to exert its effect within 1 hour. Option (a) is necessary, but assessing the client is the priority. Option (b) is important, but it will be important to inform the physician of the current blood pressure. Option (d) is a good follow-up intervention but not the priority intervention.

2. A beta-blocking agent is added to the pharmacologic therapy of a client with heart failure. An expected therapeutic effect is
   a. a decrease in complaints of fatigue.
   (b.) a decrease in the heart rate.
   c. an increase in blood pressure.
   d. an increase in diuresis.

   Rationale: The answer is (b). Beta-blockers decrease the effects of epinephrine and norepinephrine. The physiologic effect is to decrease cardiac contractibility and workload. Option (a) The client may have an increase rather than a decrease in fatigue after beginning therapy. Options (c) and (d) do not address the mechanism of action of beta-blockers.

3. The client is taking hydrochlorothiazide 25 mg po daily and is started on the ACE inhibitor lisinopril 10 mg po daily. Which nursing intervention indicates the most appropriate follow-through action?
   a. Monitor the client's output.
   b. Assess the client for impaired skin integrity.
   c. Assess the client's cardiac rhythm.
   (d.) Monitor the client's blood pressure.

   Rationale: The answer is (d). The drug combination indicates the primary use is for the antihypertensive effects. Blood pressure should be monitored before and after drug administration. Options (a), (b), and (c) do not address the effects of the combined drug therapy.

5-4 NCLEX EXAMINATION PREPARATION #4

INSTRUCTIONS: Circle the one best answer for each test question. Write your rationale for selecting the answer. To enhance your learning and test-taking skills, discuss your answer and rationale with a partner. The answer and the rationale can be found on the back of this page.

1. The home health nurse visits a client who has a history of heart failure. The client is on an ACE inhibitor, a loop diuretic, and a nitrate drug. While talking with the client, the nurse notices that the client has a persistent dry, nonproductive cough. Which nursing action is most appropriate?
   a. Ask whether the client is taking any cough medicine.
   b. Encourage the client to increase fluid intake.
   c. Ask whether the client has had any chest pain.
   d. Notify the physician.

   Rationale: _____
   _____
   _____
   _____
   _____

2. The nurse is providing discharge instructions to an elderly client taking the following oral medications: warfarin 5 mg daily, furosemide 20 mg daily, and digoxin 0.125 mg every other day. Which of the following is most important for the nurse to include in the instructions?
   a. "You can take the pills with meals."
   b. "Call the doctor if you notice any bruising."
   c. "Use a pill box to remind you of the medicines you need to take."
   d. "Take the furosemide in the morning so you can sleep at night."

   Rationale: _____
   _____
   _____
   _____
   _____

3. The nurse is delegating the care of a client who is now stable after requiring a chest tube insertion for complications related to the insertion of a central subclavian line the night before. Which intervention is most important for the nurse to ask the nursing assistant to carry out?
   a. Count the respiratory rate for 1 full minute.
   b. Keep the client in high Fowler's position.
   c. Assist the client to cough and deep breathe.
   d. Ask the client to remain in bed while the chest tube is in place.

   Rationale: _____
   _____
   _____
   _____
   _____

ANSWER KEY FOR NCLEX EXAMINATION PREPARATION #4

HELPFUL HINTS: Read all test questions carefully. Identify key words in the question that will guide you in answering the question. In these test questions the **key words** to consider are **"most appropriate"** and **"most important."** Compare your rationale with the one in the test question.

1. The home health nurse visits a client who has a history of heart failure. The client is on an ACE inhibitor, a loop diuretic, and a nitrate drug. While talking with the client, the nurse notices that the client has a persistent dry, nonproductive cough. Which nursing action is most appropriate?
   a. Ask whether the client is taking any cough medicine.
   b. Encourage the client to increase fluid intake.
   c. Ask whether the client has had any chest pain.
   (d.) Notify the physician.

   Rationale: The answer is (d). A dry, nonproductive cough is a side effect of ACE inhibitors such as enalapril. This may warrant a change in therapy. Options (a), (b), and (c) do not address this side effect.

2. The nurse is providing discharge instructions to an elderly client taking the following oral medications: warfarin 5 mg daily, furosemide 20 mg daily, and digoxin 0.125 mg every other day. Which of the following is most important for the nurse to include in the instructions?
   a. "You can take the pills with meals."
   (b.) "Call the doctor if you notice any bruising."
   c. "Use a pill box to remind you of the medicines you need to take."
   d. "Take the furosemide in the morning so you can sleep at night."

   Rationale: The answer is (b). On the basis of this situation, it is most important to teach the client to recognize signs of excessive anticoagulation therapy. Options (a) and (d) are good but not the most important. Option (c) may not be the best because mixing digoxin with the other pills may be confusing for the elderly client if the digoxin needs to be held.

3. The nurse is delegating the care of a client who is now stable after requiring a chest tube insertion for complications related to the insertion of a central subclavian line the night before. Which intervention is most important for the nurse to ask the nursing assistant to carry out?
   a. Count the respiratory rate for 1 full minute.
   b. Keep the client in high Fowler's position.
   (c.) Assist the client to cough and deep breathe.
   d. Ask the client to remain in bed while the chest tube is in place.

   Rationale: The answer is (c). Clients with chest tubes should be encouraged to cough and deep breathe to enhance lung reexpansion. Options (a) and (b) are good but not the most important. Option (d) is not appropriate, and, unless contraindicated, the client should be encouraged to ambulate.

5-5 NCLEX EXAMINATION PREPARATION #5

INSTRUCTIONS: Circle the one best answer for each test question. Write your rationale for selecting the answer. To enhance your learning and test-taking skills, discuss your answer and rationale with a partner. The answer and the rationale can be found on the back of this page.

1. The client is on a heparin infusion after being diagnosed with a venous thrombus in the right leg. To best monitor the effect of the heparin therapy, the nurse would
   a. assess for signs and symptoms of bleeding.
   b. check the aPTT.
   c. monitor the PT.
   d. check the stool for occult blood.

   Rationale: _____
   _____
   _____
   _____
   _____

2. The nurse is assigned to a client who is 4 days postop thoracic surgery and has a chest tube. The nurse learns in the morning report that there has not been any drainage from the chest tube for the last 24 hours. In assessing the closed-chest drainage system, the nurse notes that there are no fluctuations in the water-seal chamber. The client's respirations are 22, unlabored. In planning the client care, the nurse would prepare
   a. for possible chest tube removal.
   b. for replacement of the chest tube.
   c. to increase the suction to the drainage system.
   d. to disconnect the chest tube from the drainage system.

   Rationale: _____
   _____
   _____
   _____
   _____

3. An elderly client, 1 day postop right hip surgery, is confused and restless this morning. The client is receiving oxygen via a nasal cannula, has a continuous IV to gravity, and is pulling at the right hip dressing. In planning the care of the client, it is most appropriate to initially assign the
   a. staff RN to care for the client.
   b. nursing assistant to monitor the client and report changes.
   c. nursing assistant but have the RN check the client every hour.
   d. LVN/LPN to care for the client and assess for increased confusion.

   Rationale: _____
   _____
   _____
   _____
   _____

5 NCLEX Examination Preparation

ANSWER KEY FOR NCLEX EXAMINATION PREPARATION #5

HELPFUL HINTS: Read all test questions carefully. Identify key words in the question that will guide you in answering the question. In these test questions the **key words** to consider are **"best"** and **"planning the client care."** Compare your rationale with the one in the test question.

1. The client is on a heparin infusion after being diagnosed with a venous thrombus in the right leg. To best monitor the effect of the heparin therapy, the nurse would
   a. assess for signs and symptoms of bleeding.
   b. check the aPTT.
   c. monitor the PT.
   d. check the stool for occult blood.

   Rationale: The answer is (b). The aPTT (activated partial thromboplastin time) is used to monitor heparin therapy. Options (a) and (d) are good nursing interventions, but signs and symptoms are not the best indicators. Option (c) is mainly used to monitor warfarin therapy.

2. The nurse is assigned to a client who is 4 days postop thoracic surgery and has a chest tube. The nurse learns in the morning report that there has not been any drainage from the chest tube for the last 24 hours. In assessing the closed-chest drainage system, the nurse notes that there are no fluctuations in the water-seal chamber. The client's respirations are 22, unlabored. In planning the client care, the nurse would prepare
   a. for possible chest tube removal.
   b. for replacement of the chest tube.
   c. to increase the suction to the drainage system.
   d. to disconnect the chest tube from the drainage system.

   Rationale: The answer is (a). The client is 4 days postop. Respiratory signs indicate normal progression of lung reexpansion. Assessment findings do not support option (b). Options (c) and (d) demonstrate a need to review chest tubes and the drainage system.

3. An elderly client, 1 day postop right hip surgery, is confused and restless this morning. The client is receiving oxygen via a nasal cannula, has a continuous IV to gravity, and is pulling at the right hip dressing. In planning the care of the client, it is most appropriate to initially assign the
   a. staff RN to care for the client.
   b. nursing assistant to monitor the client and report changes.
   c. nursing assistant but have the RN check the client every hour.
   d. LVN/LPN to care for the client and assess for increased confusion.

   Rationale: The answer is (a). Clients whose medical condition is unstable should be assigned to the RN. The RN is the most appropriate person to assess and monitor for changes. Options (b) and (c) are not appropriate for this client who is medically unstable. Option (d) is not appropriate because it is not in the LVN/LPN scope of practice to assess clients.

5-6 NCLEX EXAMINATION PREPARATION #6

INSTRUCTIONS: Circle the best answer(s) for each test question. Write your rationale for selecting the answer. To enhance your learning and test-taking skills, discuss your answer and rationale with a partner. The answer and the rationale can be found on the back of this page.

1. The client has been on enoxaparin 30 mg subcut q12h. To implement safe care, it is most important for the nurse to (Select all that apply.):
    a. assess and report the results of the aPTT.
    b. assess and report the results of the platelet count.
    c. have available injectable protamine sulfate.
    d. have available injectable phytonadione.
    e. expel air bubble in the prefilled syringe prior to injection.

    Rationale: _____
    _____
    _____
    _____
    _____

2. The nurse is caring for a client who has a chest tube connected to a closed-chest drainage system with suction. In assessing the water-seal chamber, the nurse notes constant bubbling. Which nursing intervention is most appropriate?
    a. Record the findings.
    b. Continue to monitor the client.
    c. Check the chest tube for air leaks.
    d. Decrease the amount of suction.

    Rationale: _____
    _____
    _____
    _____
    _____

3. The nurse is totaling the chest tube output at 1400, the close of the shift. The chest tube drainage is at the 125 mL calibrated mark on the drainage device. The vertical tape along the side of the calibrated marks of the drainage device has a line drawn at 50 mL with the time of 0600. Which nursing intervention is most appropriate on the basis of this finding?
    a. Draw a line at 125 mL and indicate 1400.
    b. Document 125 mL as the output for the shift.
    c. Assess the suction chamber for patency.
    d. Strip or milk chest tube quickly for 5 to 10 seconds.

    Rationale: _____
    _____
    _____
    _____
    _____

ANSWER KEY FOR NCLEX EXAMINATION PREPARATION #6

HELPFUL HINTS: Read all test questions carefully. Identify key words in the question that will guide you in answering the question. In these test questions the **key words** to consider are **"most important"** and **"most appropriate."** Consider carefully all options in the "Select all that apply" question. Compare your rationale with the one in the test question.

1. The client has been on enoxaparin 30 mg subcut q12h. To implement safe care, it is most important for the nurse to (Select all that apply.):
   a. assess and report the results of the aPTT.
   ⓑ assess and report the results of the platelet count.
   ⓒ have available injectable protamine sulfate.
   d. have available injectable phytonadione.
   e. expel air bubble in the prefilled syringe prior to injection.

   Rationale: The answers are (b) and (c). Option (b) is correct because a decrease in the platelet count (thrombocytopenia) is an adverse side effect of enoxaparin. Option (c) is correct because injectable protamine sulfate is the antidote used when the client shows signs of bleeding related to enoxaparin. Option (a) is incorrect because aPTT is not used to monitor the effects of enoxaparin. Option (d) is incorrect because phytonadione (vitamin K) is used as an antidote for warfarin therapy. Option (e) is incorrect because loss of drug is increased when the air is expelled from the prefilled syringe.

2. The nurse is caring for a client who has a chest tube connected to a closed-chest drainage system with suction. In assessing the water-seal chamber, the nurse notes constant bubbling. Which nursing intervention is most appropriate?
   a. Record the findings.
   b. Continue to monitor the client.
   ⓒ Check the chest tube for air leaks.
   d. Decrease the amount of suction.

   Rationale: The answer is (c). Constant bubbling in the water-seal chamber indicates an air leak. Options (a) and (b) are good interventions but are not the most appropriate on the basis of the situation. Option (d) does not address the water-seal chamber.

3. The nurse is totaling the chest tube output at 1400, the close of the shift. The chest tube drainage is at the 125 mL calibrated mark on the drainage device. The vertical tape along the side of the calibrated marks of the drainage device has a line drawn at 50 mL with the time of 0600. Which nursing intervention is most appropriate on the basis of this finding?
   ⓐ Draw a line at 125 mL and indicate 1400.
   b. Document 125 mL as the output for the shift.
   c. Assess the suction chamber for patency.
   d. Strip or milk chest tube quickly for 5 to 10 seconds.

   Rationale: The answer is (a). The nurse monitors the chest tube drainage output by drawing a line at the drainage level in the chamber at the end of the shift. Option (b) does not reflect the correct chest tube drainage for the shift, which is 75 mL. Option (c) is not an appropriate intervention, and option (d) is not standard nursing practice when caring for clients with chest tubes.

5-7 NCLEX EXAMINATION PREPARATION #7

INSTRUCTIONS: Circle the one best answer for each test question. Write your rationale for selecting the answer. To enhance your learning and test-taking skills, discuss your answer and rationale with a partner. The answer and the rationale can be found on the back of this page.

1. The nurse assesses the client who is 1 day postop transurethral resection of the prostate. He has not had any output from the urinary catheter for 2 hours. The client has an order for intermittent manual bladder irrigation. Which technique is best for the nurse to use to safely carry out this order?
   a. Irrigate with 50 mL of sterile water and aspirate an equal amount of fluid.
   b. Use clean technique and irrigate until the return is free of clots.
   c. Use sterile technique and irrigate with 50 mL of solution at a time.
   d. Start continuous bladder irrigation and infuse 200 mL over 30 minutes.

   Rationale: _____
   _____
   _____
   _____
   _____

2. The client has just had a generalized tonic-clonic–type seizure in bed. Which nursing intervention is of priority immediately after the seizure?
   a. Record the findings.
   b. Maintain a quiet environment.
   c. Reorient the client to the surroundings.
   d. Position the client in a side-lying position.

   Rationale: _____
   _____
   _____
   _____
   _____

3. The nurse is assigned to a client who is 4 days postop right hip replacement. The nurse finds the client eating breakfast, sitting comfortably in a chair with the right leg crossed over the left leg. Which nursing intervention is of priority?
   a. Assess the right hip dressing.
   b. Assess the client's pain level.
   c. Check the quality of the pedal pulses of both feet.
   d. Instruct the client to keep both feet flat on the floor.

   Rationale: _____
   _____
   _____
   _____
   _____

ANSWER KEY FOR NCLEX EXAMINATION PREPARATION #7

HELPFUL HINTS: Read all test questions carefully. Identify key words in the question that will guide you in answering the question. In these test questions the **key words** to consider are **"best"** and **"priority."** Compare your rationale with the one in the test question.

1. The nurse assesses the client who is 1 day postop transurethral resection of the prostate. He has not had any output from the urinary catheter for 2 hours. The client has an order for intermittent manual bladder irrigation. Which technique is best for the nurse to use to safely carry out this order?
   a. Irrigate with 50 mL of sterile water and aspirate an equal amount of fluid.
   b. Use clean technique and irrigate until the return is free of clots.
   (c.) Use sterile technique and irrigate with 50 mL of solution at a time.
   d. Start continuous bladder irrigation and infuse 200 mL over 30 minutes.

   Rationale: The answer is (c). Bladder irrigation is always performed with sterile technique. Solution is gently introduced into the bladder during irrigation. Options (a), (b), and (d) do not describe how to safely and correctly carry out this technique.

2. The client has just had a generalized tonic-clonic–type seizure in bed. Which nursing intervention is of priority immediately after the seizure?
   a. Record the findings.
   b. Maintain a quiet environment.
   c. Reorient the client to the surroundings.
   (d.) Position the client in a side-lying position.

   Rationale: The answer is (d). Aspiration is a concern after the seizure because the client will be lethargic and oral secretions will need to be suctioned and allowed to drain. Options (a), (b), and (c) are good interventions but are not the priority.

3. The nurse is assigned to a client who is 4 days postop right hip replacement. The nurse finds the client eating breakfast, sitting comfortably in a chair with the right leg crossed over the left leg. Which nursing intervention is of priority?
   a. Assess the right hip dressing.
   b. Assess the client's pain level.
   c. Check the quality of the pedal pulses of both feet.
   (d.) Instruct the client to keep both feet flat on the floor.

   Rationale: The answer is (d). Crossing of the feet or legs after hip replacement may put undue tension on the operative hip and increase the risk of hip dislocation. Options (a) and (c) are good interventions but not the priority interventions. Option (b) is important; initial client observation indicates that client is eating and sitting comfortably.

5-8 NCLEX EXAMINATION PREPARATION #8

INSTRUCTIONS: Circle the one best answer for each test question. Write your rationale for selecting the answer. To enhance your learning and test-taking skills, discuss your answer and rationale with a partner. The answer and the rationale can be found on the back of this page.

1. The client is 4 days postop colon resection and has an NG tube to low continuous suction. The client tells the nurse that he is feeling nauseated and then vomits 100 mL of yellow-green drainage. The nurse's initial action is to
    a. assess tube placement and patency.
    b. administer an antiemetic.
    c. pull out the NG tube.
    d. increase the NG tube suction to moderate.

    Rationale: _____
    _____
    _____

2. The client has been on full-strength formula tube feeding at 60 mL/hr through the NG tube for 2 days. In delegating the care of the client, which directive given to the nursing assistant most indicates that the nurse is monitoring for tube feeding complications?
    a. "Let me know if the client has liquid bowel movements this shift."
    b. "Weigh the client on the stand-up scale as soon as report is over."
    c. "The client can sit in a chair for 30 minutes this morning."
    d. "Take the vital signs every 4 hours."

    Rationale: _____
    _____
    _____

3. The nurse was assigned to a patient with a chest tube on the 0700–1500 shift. The nurse marks the level of the chest tube drainage at 1400 on the chest tube drainage device. In the electronic health record, it is most important for the nurse to document the chest tube drainage as
    a. 100 mL.
    b. 90 mL.
    c. 50 mL.
    d. 40 mL.

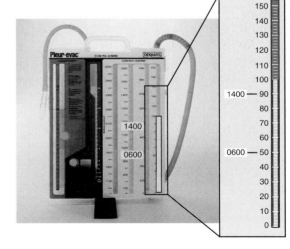

    Rationale: _____
    _____
    _____

ANSWER KEY FOR NCLEX EXAMINATION PREPARATION #8

HELPFUL HINTS: Read all test questions carefully. Identify key words in the question that will guide you in answering the question. In these test questions the **key words** to consider are **"initial," "most indicates,"** and **"most important."** Compare your rationale with the one in the test question.

1. The client is 4 days postop colon resection and has an NG tube to low continuous suction. The client tells the nurse that he is feeling nauseated and then vomits 100 mL of yellow-green drainage. The nurse's initial action is to
   a. assess tube placement and patency.
   b. administer an antiemetic.
   c. pull out the NG tube.
   d. increase the NG tube suction to moderate.

   Rationale: The answer is (a). It is important to check the placement and patency of the NG tube and ensure that the suction is working. Option (b) may be performed if the nausea and vomiting do not subside, but should not be the initial action. Options (c) and (d) do not help to solve the problem.

2. The client has been on full-strength formula tube feeding at 60 mL/hr through the NG tube for 2 days. In delegating the care of the client, which directive given to the nursing assistant most indicates that the nurse is monitoring for tube feeding complications?
   a. "Let me know if the client has liquid bowel movements this shift."
   b. "Weigh the client on the stand-up scale as soon as report is over."
   c. "The client can sit in a chair for 30 minutes this morning."
   d. "Take the vital signs every 4 hours."

   Rationale: The answer is (a). Enteral feeding formulas can cause diarrhea. Option (b) helps to identify whether the client is gaining weight. Options (c) and (d) are directives that promote good nursing care, but they are not directly related to identifying the effects related to full-strength formula tube feedings.

3. The nurse was assigned to a patient with a chest tube on the 0700–1500 shift. The nurse marks the level of the chest tube drainage at 1400 on the chest tube drainage device. In the electronic health record, it is most important for the nurse to document the chest tube drainage as:
   a. 100 mL.
   b. 90 mL.
   c. 50 mL.
   d. 40 mL.

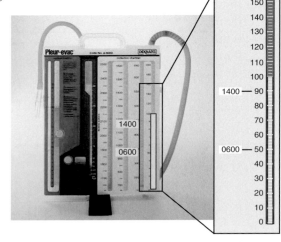

   Rationale: The answer is (d). The chest tube drainage at 0600 was 50 mL. At 1400 the drainage is at the 90 mL calibrated marking (90 mL – 50 mL = 40 mL). Options (a), (b), and (c) are incorrect in reading the calibrated drainage from the chest tube drainage device.

Professional Nursing Practice

6-1 QUALITY NURSING PRACTICE SITUATION #1 (POSTSURGICAL PATIENT)

Patient Plan of Care		
Lab/Diagnostic Tests	**Medications**	
ECG ☑	Ketorolac 10 mg IM q6h ×24 hr Acetaminophen #3 tab i po q3h prn pain Metoclopramide 10 mg IVP q6h prn N/V	Diet: Clear liquid – DAT
	Indwelling urinary catheter	VS q4h Antiembolic stockings Seq. compression device	Ambulate with assistance Incentive spirometer q2h
	IV Fluids: 1 L lactated Ringer's q8h	
Name: CJ	Age: 60 Full code	Dx: Prostate cancer Surg: Robotic prostatectomy

Morning handoff report: "The patient is 1 day postop. He was possibly being discharged today, but he had some chest pain last night and I heard fine crackles on the right lower lung base. Bowel sounds are faint in the four quadrants. Vital signs are stable. Pain level 2. The urinary catheter is patent, draining blood-tinged urine. Please encourage the patient to use the incentive spirometer and have him ambulate more today. An ECG was done last night. His doctor will be in sometime this morning."

Using Nursing Knowledge

Based on the morning handoff report and the Patient Plan of Care, answer the following:

- List assessment priorities:

  _____
  _____
  _____

- Identify the priorities of the plan of care for the morning:

  _____
  _____

- List signs and symptoms that might indicate possible complications that the nurse should monitor and include in the plan of care:

  _____
  _____
  _____

Using Leadership Skills

Consider the scope of practice and then determine the nursing interventions that may be delegated to the:

LVN/LPN:

_____
_____
_____
_____
_____

Unlicensed nursing assistant:

_____
_____
_____

Evidence-Based Practice

Use appropriate resources to answer the following question:
In clients who have a radical prostatectomy, how effective is the robotic surgical method in enhancing postop recovery compared with clients who have a transurethral resection of the prostate?

_____
_____

6 Professional Nursing Practice

Review the following diagram, "Caring for the Whole Person." Use the boxes to

1. identify **actual and potential** concerns related to the social needs of the client.
2. identify the **physiologic** needs at discharge.
3. list **individual considerations** for the client on discharge.

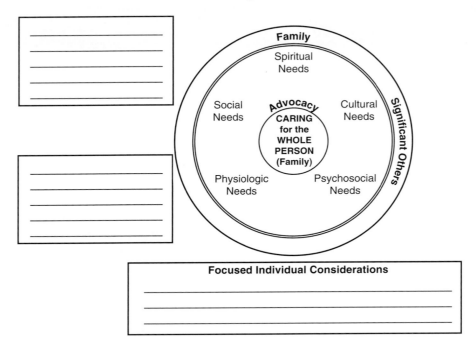

Focused Individual Considerations
_____
_____
_____

⚙ **Collaborative Learning Activity:** With a partner, use the textbooks and information from appropriate websites to answer and complete the possible discharge instructions for the client:

Possible discharge instructions:

Regarding Urinary Catheter: _____
_____
_____

Discharge Medications: _____
_____
_____

Activity: _____
_____

Follow-up Visit: _____
_____

Potential Complications: _____
_____
_____

6-2 QUALITY NURSING PRACTICE SITUATION #2 (CARING AND ADVOCACY)

Patient Plan of Care		
Lab/Diagnostic Tests	**Medications**	
FBG in AM Electrolyte panel in AM UA ☐	Lorazepam 0.5 mg IV stat	Diet: Mech soft NPO p̄ midnight
	O_2 per NC @ 3 L/min	VS, pulse ox q4h and prn I & O q shift Bed rest
IV Fluids: 1 L 0.9% sodium chloride at 50 mL/hr		
Name: SP Age: 75	Full code	Dx: Acute confusion

Evening Handoff Report at 2300: "The client was admitted from the emergency department around 1900. The wife says that she noticed that her husband started to get confused last evening. The wife, who is 70 yrs old, has been with him all day and looks very tired. She is waiting for her son to pick her up but does not really want to leave her husband. She says they have been married 50 years and they rarely have been separated from each other. The admitting orders are on the chart. I gave him lorazepam IV for restlessness at 2100. The wife says he has been taking zolpidem for sleep. You might want to call the doctor for an order of zolpidem if the lorazepam does not calm him down. The latest VS are T 99.6°F, P 92 irregular, R 18 shallow, BP 136/90, pulse ox 94% on oxygen at 3 L/min. Unable to determine if the patient is having pain since he does not respond appropriately to the pain assessment scale."

Using Nursing Knowledge
Based on the evening report and Patient Plan of Care, answer the following:

• List assessment priorities:

_____

_____

• Identify the priorities of the plan of care for the shift:

_____

_____

_____

_____

• List signs and symptoms that might indicate possible complications that the nurse should monitor and include in the plan of care:

_____

_____

Using Leadership Skills
Consider the scope of practice, then determine the nursing interventions that may be delegated for this client to the:

LVN/LPN:

_____

_____

_____

_____

Unlicensed nursing assistant:

_____

_____

_____

Evidence-Based Practice
Use appropriate resources to answer the following question:
In elderly clients aged 75 years and older, is lorazepam effective in decreasing anxiety and restlessness?

_____

_____

6 Professional Nursing Practice

Review the following diagram, "Caring for the Whole Person." Use the boxes to

1. identify <u>**actual and potential physiologic**</u> concerns related to the care of the client.
2. identify the <u>**actual or potential psychosocial**</u> concerns expressed by the <u>wife</u>.
3. list **individual considerations** for the care of the client.

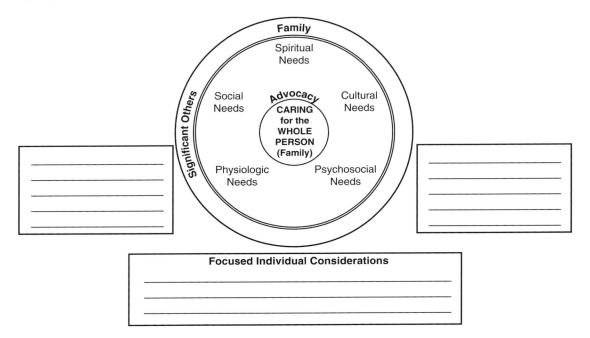

Collaborative Learning Activity: With a partner, use the following part of the clinical situation to write possible therapeutic communication statements that demonstrate caring and advocacy:

The wife, who is 70 years old, has been with him all day and looks very tired. She is waiting for her son to pick her up but does not really want to leave her husband. She says they have been married 50 years and they rarely have been separated from each other.

Write possible therapeutic communication statements that demonstrate **caring:**

_____
_____
_____
_____
_____
_____
_____

Write a possible therapeutic communication statement that demonstrates **advocacy:**

_____
_____
_____
_____

6 Professional Nursing Practice

6-3 QUALITY NURSING PRACTICE SITUATION #3 (ADVERSE CLIENT OUTCOME)

Patient Plan of Care

Medications

Amlodipine 5 mg po daily
Cimetidine 400 mg po QID
Glyburide 2.5 mg po daily
Nitroglycerin 0.4 mg SL i tab q5min ×3 prn chest pain

Diet: 1800 ADA

FSBG qAM & qPM
(Call MD if greater than 150 mg/dL)
O_2 per NC @ 3 L/min prn

VS q4h
I & O
Up in chair tid
Antiembolic hose

Saline lock flush with NS q shift

Name: RA Age: 60	Full code	Dx: Pneumonia, hypertension Hx of CAD, unstable angina DM type 2

Handoff Report at 0700: "The client had a restful night. He says he is going home this morning. His lungs are clear and the vital signs are stable with a BP of 140/88. He complained of some indigestion a little while ago, so I gave the cimetidine early. Aside from his routine medications and removal of his saline lock on discharge, he is ready to go."

Progression of Adverse Outcome
- After report the RN visits the client and asks the client whether the cimetidine has helped him. The client says it was just given to him so that it will take a few more minutes for the drug to work. He asks for the emesis basin "just in case."
- The RN asks the certified nursing assistant to take the pulse and BP because the client is diaphoretic. Dynamap readings indicate an increase in pulse and a BP of 120/70.
- The RN asks the LVN to start the oxygen and asks the CNA to take vital signs q5min.
- The RN goes to call the physician.
- Ten minutes later the LVN calls a code. After 30 minutes of CPR the client is pronounced dead.

Using Leadership Skills
List the current needs that are associated with the care of the family experiencing the death of a loved one:
- Prepare for family visit (Who should be involved?)
- Postdeath care can be done by:
- Notify pastoral care (Who should notify?)
- Document (Who should document?)

Evaluate the situation:
What could have been done differently?

6 Professional Nursing Practice

Evidence-Based Practice
Use appropriate resources to answer the following question:
In acute care settings that have rapid response teams, are nursing staff from noncritical care units consistently utilizing the rapid response team for patients who are clinically deteriorating?

Review the following diagram, "Caring for the Whole Person." Use the boxes to

1. identify __actual and potential__ psychosocial needs for the __family__ related to the unexpected death of the client.
2. list **individual considerations** for the postdeath care of the client.

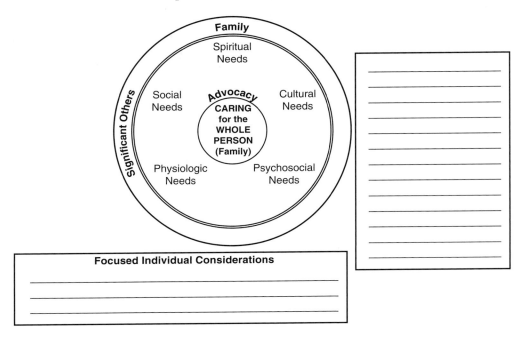

Focused Individual Considerations

_____

_____

_____

Collaborative Learning Activity: With a partner, reread the situation. Discuss and answer the following:

• If you are the **staff nurse,** what could have been done differently?

_____

_____

_____

• If you are the **staff nurse,** what would be most helpful now after reviewing and experiencing the adverse event?

_____

_____

_____

• If you are the **unit supervisor,** what could have been done differently?

_____

_____

_____

• If you are the **unit supervisor,** what would be most helpful for the staff nurse? Unit? Hospital?

_____

_____

_____

6 Professional Nursing Practice

7-1 WORKING WITH PHARMACOLOGY #1

Instructions: Read the mini scenario, and from your knowledge of pharmacology, fill in the drug classification for the drug identified in the scenario. All of the listed **side effects/adverse effects** are associated with the drug. Research the side effect/adverse effect that is highlighted with a (●) using appropriate resources.
- Write the research findings.
- Identify patient instructions related to this drug therapy.

The nurse is caring for a patient who has been taking atorvastatin 20 mg po BID for 2 months to lower cholesterol levels. **Drug classification:**	Side effects/adverse effects of this drug: • Headache • Dizziness • Muscle pain ● • Abdominal cramps • Skin rash	Research findings:
The nurse is caring for a patient who has been taking propranolol 80 mg po q8h to control an irregular heartbeat. **Drug classification:**	Side effects/adverse effects of this drug: • Slow pulse ● • Dizziness • Weakness • Impotence • Skin rash	Research findings:
The nurse is caring for a patient who has been taking phenytoin 200 mg po q8h for a seizure disorder. **Drug classification:**	Side effects/adverse effects of this drug: • Diplopia • Nystagmus • Weight loss • Swollen gums • Agranulocytosis ●	Research findings:

7-2 WORKING WITH PHARMACOLOGY #2

Instructions: Read the mini scenario, and from your knowledge of pharmacology, fill in the drug classification for the drug identified in the scenario. All of the listed **side effects/adverse effects** are associated with the drug. Research the side effect/adverse effect that is highlighted with a (●) using appropriate resources.

- Write the research findings.
- Identify patient instructions related to this drug therapy.

The nurse is assessing a patient who has been taking prednisone 10 mg po daily for 2 months for Crohn disease. Drug classification:	Side effects/adverse effects of this drug: • Mood swings • Ecchymosis • Anorexia • Stomach pain ● • Restlessness	Research findings:
The nurse is administering ketorolac 10 mg IM q6h to a postsurgical patient. Drug classification:	Side effects/adverse effects of this drug: • Drowsiness • Paresthesia • Abdominal pain ● • Dyspepsia • Urinary frequency	Research findings:
The nurse is assessing a patient who is on clopidogrel 75 mg po daily after suffering a recent stroke. Drug classification:	Side effects/adverse effects of this drug: • Nose bleed • Neutropenia ● • Depression • Headache • Diarrhea	Research findings:

7-3 WORKING WITH PHARMACOLOGY #3

Instructions: Read the mini scenario, and from your knowledge of pharmacology, fill in the drug classification for the drug identified in the scenario. All of the listed **side effects/adverse effects** are associated with the drug. Research the side effect/adverse effect that is highlighted with a (●) using appropriate resources.

- Write the research findings.
- Identify patient instructions related to this drug therapy.

The nurse administers lorazepam 4 mg IVP as a preop medication to a patient. Drug classification:	Side effects/adverse effects of this drug: • Dizziness • Dyspnea ● • Lethargy • Depression • Drowsiness	Research findings:
The nurse is preparing the 0900 dose of captopril 50 mg po for the patient diagnosed with heart failure. Drug classification:	Side effects/adverse effects of this drug: • Fatigue • Headache • Nonproductive cough • Neutropenia ● • Dizziness	Research findings:
The nurse is assessing a patient who has atrial fibrillation and is on digoxin 0.25 mg po daily. Drug classification:	Side effects/adverse effects of this drug: • Dysrhythmia ● • Fatigue • Yellow vision • Abdominal pain • Headache	Research findings:

7 Evaluation

7-4 WORKING WITH PHARMACOLOGY #4

Instructions: Read the mini scenario, and from your knowledge of pharmacology, fill in the drug classification for the drug identified in the scenario. All of the listed **side effects/adverse effects** are associated with the drug. Research the side effect/adverse effect that is highlighted with a (●) using appropriate resources.
- Write the research findings.
- Identify patient instructions related to this drug therapy.

The nurse is administering levo-floxacin 500 mg IVPB daily to a patient post-operatively. **Drug classification:**	**Side effects/adverse effects of this drug:** • Dizziness • Insomnia • Abdominal pain • Diarrhea • Tendon pain ●	**Research findings:**
The nurse is teaching a patient how to use a metaproterenol sulfate inhaler and signs and symptoms related to use. **Drug classification:**	**Side effects/adverse effects of this drug:** • Nervousness • Headache • Difficulty breathing ● • Fine hand tremors • Restlessness	**Research findings:**
The patient is started on vanco-mycin 500 mg IVPB in 100 mL 0.9% NaCl daily. **Drug classification:**	**Side effects/adverse effects of this drug:** • Phlebitis • Flushing of face/torso ● • Nausea • Headache • Diarrhea	**Research findings:**

7-5 WORKING WITH DECISION MAKING

Instructions: Read the mini scenario found in the box. Then decide whether the clinical decision, action, or intervention made by the nurse was appropriate. Provide a rationale for your decision.

Situation #1	Clinical Decision/Action/Intervention
The nurse is caring for a patient who has been diagnosed with diabetes mellitus type 1. The patient is started on insulin glargine 26 units daily in the evening and a correction insulin scale (sliding scale) with regular insulin. The nurse provides the following instructions to the patient: 1. Insulin glargine is a long-acting insulin that is administered once a day, usually in the evening. 2. Regular insulin may be combined with insulin glargine in the same insulin syringe if your fingerstick blood glucose results indicate the need for regular insulin coverage.	☐ **Appropriate** ☐ **Not Appropriate** **Rationale:**

Situation #2	Clinical Decision/Action/Intervention
The nurse is caring for a patient diagnosed with a DVT. An IV of 1000 mL 0.9% NaCl with heparin 20,000 units is started and the physician orders for the patient to receive 500 units of heparin per hour. The nurse sets the IV pump at 32 mL/hr. Has the nurse carried out the order correctly?	☐ **Appropriate** ☐ **Not Appropriate** **Rationale:**

Situation #3	Clinical Decision/Action/Intervention
The RN is working with a staff LVN during the weekend. Throughout the shift, the RN delegates the following nursing interventions to the LVN: 1. Monitor a blood transfusion. 2. Start an IV of lactated Ringer's solution. 3. Collect a sterile UA specimen via a straight catheterization. 4. Admit a new patient. 5. Administer nitroglycerin SL to a patient experiencing angina.	☐ **Appropriate** ☐ **Not Appropriate** **Rationale:**

7-6 WORKING WITH PRIORITY SETTING

Instructions: Read the Patient Plan of Care and the nursing notes gathered from the night shift on client RM.

Diagnostic Tests	Routine Medications	
Na⁺, K⁺, Cl⁻, BUN	Furosemide 20 mg IVP 0900	Diet: 1800 Cal ADA NAS
CBC today (10/8)	Metformin 500 mg po BID	Bed rest with BRP
FBG today (10/8)	Docusate 100 mg po qAM Temazepam 7.5 mg po tab i at bedtime if needed	LBM: 10/06 VS routine
IV Pyelogram today (10/8)	Saline lock inserted 10/05	Fingerstick BG qAM (0730) & qPM (1700)
	Sliding scale insulin coverage: 200–175 give 3 units regular insulin 174–150 give 2 units regular insulin 149–125 no insulin	I & O
		Chg Ⓛ leg dressing q shift
		Elevate leg on pillow

Pt. Name: RM   Age: 66   Admitted: 10/4   Rm: 255   Dx: Cellulitis left leg/DM type 2

Date	Time	Nurse's Notes
10/08	0100	Awake, states is worried about the infection in his leg. Left leg elevated on pillow. Dressing dry and intact, no drainage noted. Requested sleeping medication. Medicated with temazepam 7.5 mg.
	0200	Sleeping
	0600	Awake, small amount of serosanguineous drainage noted on dressing. C/o leg pain 5/10 on the pain scale, states "wants to wait to see if the pain goes away in a few minutes." Fasting blood glucose was drawn this morning.

Instructions: Based on your evaluation of the Patient Plan of Care and the Nurse's Notes, (1) complete the clinical worksheet with your notes for the required care and (2) list your priority nursing actions.

Clinical Worksheet	List Priority Nursing Actions
Pt. Name: _____ Room: _____ Dx: _____ VS: _____ at _____ Drg chg ( ) Saline lock ( ) I & O ( ) Elevate leg on pillow ( ) Medications: _____ _____ _____ _____ _____ _____	